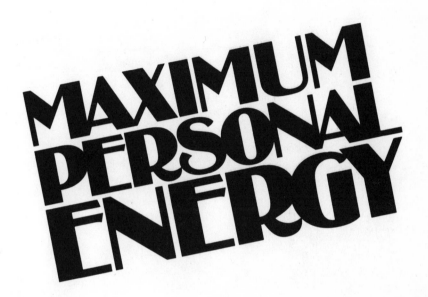

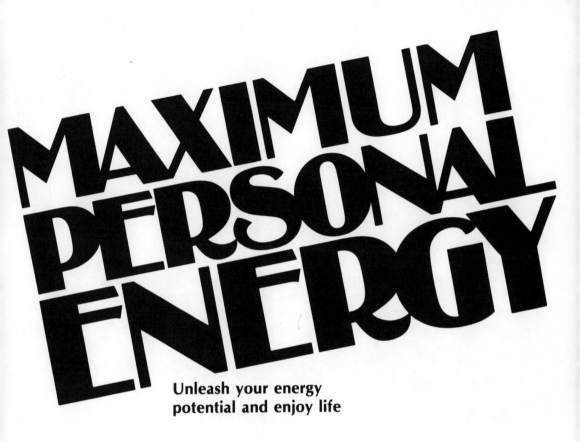

MAXIMUM PERSONAL ENERGY

Unleash your energy
potential and enjoy life

by Charles T. Kuntzleman, Ed.D.

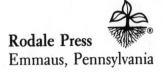

Rodale Press
Emmaus, Pennsylvania

Printed in the United States of America on recycled paper, containing a high percentage of de-inked fiber.

Book design and illustrations by Barbara Field

Library of Congress Cataloging in Publication Data

Kuntzleman, Charles T.
    Maximum personal energy.

    Includes index.
    1. Vitality. 2. Health. I. Title.
RA776.5.K85   613   81-10702
ISBN 0-87857-364-X (hardcover) AACR2
ISBN 0-87857-363-1 (paperback)

2   4   6   8   10   9   7   5   3   1   hardcover
2   4   6   8   10   9   7   5   3   1   paperback

Table of Contents

Acknowledgments

Authors have many people to thank when writing a book. This book is no exception. I'm particularly indebted to Lyn Cryderman and Dan Runyon for editorial assistance, research, and pertinent recommendations on *Maximum Personal Energy*'s content, style, and organization. Dan Wallace, my editor at Rodale Press, helped with many editorial suggestions that greatly improved the quality of the book. An additional word of thanks goes to Lynette Van Alstine, my ever-efficient secretary, who typed and retyped the manuscript and then patiently made all the changes that I wanted after I promised "this is the last time."

Beth deserves a gold medal for patience, support, and understanding. Only a spouse knows the sacrifices that must be made when working on a book, especially during the last month. Finally, I am particularly grateful to the many health, energy, and fitness experts whose work and insight I used to make this book a reality. Thank you all.

Prologue

For almost 20 years now I've been trying to help people live well. I've traveled over the United States, Canada, and Europe conducting fitness, nutrition, weight control, and general well-being workshops. I've passed out advice to physicians, corporate executives, hospital administrators, educators, church leaders, Young Men's Christian Association (YMCA) personnel, and anyone else that I suspected might be willing to listen to me. I've tried to convince them to help themselves to a better life and then have them convince others to do the same.

I also listened carefully to what people were saying to me. I noticed that most people didn't talk about improving their health. Instead, they talked about increasing their energy levels. They were interested in having more bounce to the ounce—more get-up-and-go. I vividly recall one woman telling me, "I'm so low on the energy scale that the best part of the day is over when my alarm clock goes off."

The problems were not just individual; they were corporate. Industrial and educational leaders told me that if I could get their people out of their doldrums, get them moving again and feeling more energetic, I would make a significant improvement in the success and productivity of their organization.

Intrigued, I started to explore this phenomenon of energy. First, I searched for a good definition of energy. I cornered a nuclear engineer and asked him. He told me that, to him, energy is the binding force in the nucleus of an atom. Not satisfied, I talked to a physicist, who explained that energy is the capacity for doing work and overcoming resistance. A physiologist defined energy as your body's capacity for doing work. And a nutritionist I interviewed insisted that energy is a chemical reaction that takes place in your body as food is digested, assimilated, and used. A weight-control expert said energy is the amount of calories expended for a particular activity, or the amount of energy units inherent in a selected food, while a yogi told me that energy was the force, the power, within us all.

They were good answers and I liked them all. So I put them together as a definition of energy. Energy is your zest for working, playing, loving—living. It is the biological power or force within you—your physical capacity for living and your mental attitude toward your capacity for living. In practical terms, you have "energy" if you can get through your working day with enough resources to meet unexpected demands, and still enjoy life.

It's funny. We all know when we have energy. We have felt its rush when taking a walk in the crisp, fall air; upon receiving a hard-earned promotion or raise; anticipating Christmas morning; or reacting to a dangerous situation such as a near car accident. With the rush we become acutely alert, vibrant, and quick-thinking. Life is exciting. Sleep or drowsiness has no place.

While I was trying to put this elusive definition of energy together, I turned the question around and asked the average person on the street what energy wasn't. "That's when I feel pooped out . . . tired," came the average response. But perhaps the most graphic was the matronly school teacher who told me that lack of energy is when you sit in a rocking chair and can't get it going. We know when we don't have it—the drowsiness after a big meal; the fatigue after hours of Christmas shopping; the unresponsiveness on a hot humid afternoon. We understand those fatigues. What really concerns us is the burn-out some of us feel. We enter employment full of great enthusiasm and vigor, but before the task is completed we notice in ourselves a waning of interest and a lack of drive and desire.

Why? To find the answer I became an observer of human nature. I tried to find out what makes some people more energetic than others. Why are some people energizers while other people seem to get winded dialing long-distance phone numbers? The more I observed, the more it became apparent that energetic people have certain common characteristics. Also, while energy levels vary from person to person, the true energizers are maximizing their energy potentials.

Their characteristics? Energizing people tend to be more fit, eat better foods, are relatively slim, enjoy life, handle change well, get along well with their counterparts, and have a strong sense of control and direction in their lives. They understand that it is their individual responsibility to improve their energy levels and not to depend on external sources such as cigarettes, alcohol, drugs, or excessive caffeine.

I don't want you to get the impression that I've got everything knocked. Personally, I've been working on all these things myself. I'm growing as an individual, trying to develop my own levels of maximum personal energy. I believe very strongly in the system outlined on these pages and have seen dramatic results occur in many, many people.

As you read this book, you will find some things that apply directly to your situation, while other areas may seem somewhat unrelated to your present lifestyle. I encourage you to select those things which seem to be related to your present condition and apply them to your day-to-day routines. If you give them a chance, they will work.

You probably know some high-energy people yourself. They are full of vigor, drive, and a love for living. If you watch, analyze, and question them, you'll find that they have many of the characteristics I've mentioned. Such people will tell you there aren't any pat answers to maximum personal energy. I agree. But there are steps that you can take to help improve your energy level. And that's what this book is all about. Although the guidelines I have provided are simple, following them is not. But it can be done with a lot less effort than you might think. And I am confident that you will find the results energizing.

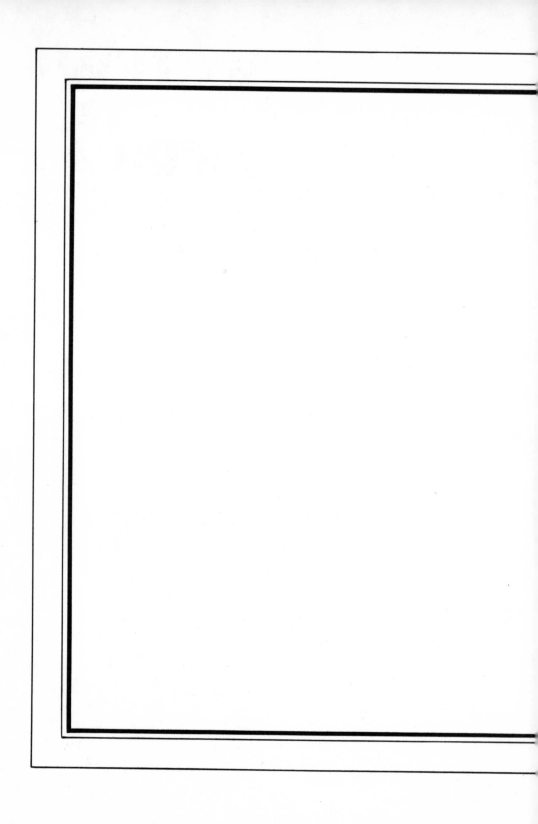

SECTION I: THE AMERICAN WAY

CHAPTER 1
Change: Prelude to Stress

A few years ago, the roof of the Kemper Arena in Kansas City collapsed. Fortunately, the 7,000-ton concrete and steel cover came down when the building was unoccupied and no one was injured. While the dust was still settling a special team of "structural detectives" arrived on the scene and they began climbing around the rubble. Some three months after the mishap the team had analyzed the data and announced the cause of the spectacular accident: stress. One giant steel bolt responsible for connecting a massive girder to another one had simply broken under stress.

It doesn't take a team of detectives to discover that the same thing is happening to a majority of the North American people. Surveys indicate that anywhere from 70 to 90 percent of us are plagued by high levels of stress. The "rat race" is no longer a joke, but a frightful reality to most of us. More and more of us, either by necessity or by choice, are falling into the trap of trying to cram 25 hours into an already cramped 24-hour day and taking on more and more responsibility with less and less time.

Homes once characterized as harmonious harbors of family dinners and congenial repartee have become "dispatch centers" for parents trying to wrestle with two jobs while shuffling their children to Little League, day care, scouts, dance class, and church. Even our churches, in campaigning for family stability and orderliness, vie for our time by offering us weeknight activities and weekend seminars on life enrichment.

Early in our history as a nation, many of us enjoyed the physical comfort of a large home surrounded by a few acres of quiet countryside, an environment that changed little, if at all. Home was a place where people held similar values and beliefs, and an environment that gave people a sense of security and stability.

But times have changed. As the population swelled and we became more industrial, people started to move to the city. Since 1940, the majority of Americans have lived in the city. According to the 1980 census, well over 70 percent of us are urban dwellers who live on 2 percent of the land. Crowded together, we compete for jobs and agonize over food and fuel shortages and skyrocketing prices. We must cope with noise, traffic jams, polluted air and water, and other headaches from increasing population density. Moreover, our private lives are becoming increasingly unstable, for the nuclear family of husband, wife, and a few children that was the norm in preindustrial societies is breaking down. In 1980, one in every five Americans lived alone. An estimated ⅔ to ¾ of our population no longer fits within the traditional pattern of nuclear family life. Roughly 40 percent of all marriages consummated today will end in divorce. And many who remain married do so only for financial and social purposes and not for a commitment to similar goals and purposes.

The rapid rate at which our society experiences change is one of the primary reasons why our levels of stress are so high. Things are moving so fast that we just can't keep up with them. And there's no getting around it. In today's world, you simply cannot escape change. We are in the midst of what Alvin Toffler calls "future shock." Future shock occurs because you are unsure. Unsure about what will happen tomorrow, next year, in ten years. You can't be sure because you're right in the midst of rapid change.

Think of some of the changes that have occurred in the past 30 years. I consider myself a young man. Most men who turn 40 do. Yet in my lifetime I went from listening to "The Green Hornet" on the radio to watching a man walk on the surface of the moon. My dad used to take me down to the airport to see the first Lockheeds, which could cross the continent in 12 hours. I was impressed. It took three days by train. Now, I have to cope with breakfast on the plane in Chicago, only to get off the plane in Los Angeles and be taken out to breakfast. The first time I ever filled up my gas tank, a man came out in a white shirt and black bow tie, filled the tank, checked the oil, cleaned the front and back windows and gave me a free roadmap; all for 19.9¢ a gallon. Now, when I want gasoline, I pump it myself and pay the attendant through a bullet-proof window, for $1.25 a gallon.

Surprisingly, even pleasant changes can produce levels of stress that can be immobilizing. Working with 5,000 patients in a special project, researchers from the University of Washington School of Medicine found that changes in an individual's lifestyle were often accompanied by changes in health. Although major life changes such as the death of a spouse, getting a divorce, or spending time in jail have the biggest impact, even desirable changes such as marriage, retirement, or an outstanding personal achievement may create stress. These clusters of life changes are cumulative, and gradually build up to the point that they amount to "life crises." Such a crisis can lower your energy levels and make you feel utterly washed out, too tired to do a thing.

Contributing to the problem is the fact that our changing culture is causing us to suffer from an identity crisis because of the way things have changed. There was a time when everyone knew their place. Either you were a peasant or a prince; a lowly dirt farmer or a land baron; a chimney sweep or a scholar. And it was easy to tell who was what. Whether it was good or bad, everyone knew their place, and they stayed put.

Today we've got millionaires' kids running around in frazzled blue jeans, daughters of paupers primping for proms, and "shop rats" tooling the town in sports cars. Merely looking in the mirror doesn't tell you who you are. This is the result of industrialization. It's a new thing under the sun that a man with an ounce of ambition who channels it properly soon can be bringing a six-figure income home (to a very fine home indeed).

At one time churches held tremendous influence and sway over their members. The priest, pastor, or church board literally dictated how people were to act. If someone stepped out of line they were severely chastised. Now, church members and leaders can't agree on the order of worship, let alone abortion, war, gay rights, and birth control. Additionally, people in the same community tended to hold similar values and beliefs. More often than not, they were from the same ethnic background—Jewish, Polish, Slavic, and the like. So political, social, educational, and religious values were the same. But today, the mobility of society, television, and the emergence of intermarrying of various ethnic groups have helped to produce confusion—true future shock.

Because of these changes, people are constantly off-guard, uncomfortable, and unsure. Values and beliefs are ill-defined. In order to survive, people must continually adapt to change. It's pervasive and inescapable, which, of course, means that the accompanying stress is impossible to avoid. In fact, efforts to avoid stress often produce more stress.

According to Dr. Hans Selye, the world's leading authority on stress, the absence of stress is death. I know that statement seems strange, but what he's really saying is that stress is essential for life. Stress makes you enjoy life. What is necessary is a balance, and an understanding that stress should be changed to a positive rather than a negative force.

Even people who seem to have it made experience stress. Nursing home directors will tell you that one of the biggest problems they face is helping their residents cope with stress, even though all of their needs are apparently met. The reason for this is change. The nursing home represents an entirely different lifestyle than what the residents have been accustomed to. For the same reasons, people who try to get away from it all often find their stress has followed them to that remote cabin or island retreat. As long as you are living, you will have stress, and chances are, tomorrow will bring you more stress than you had today.

Initially, all this may sound pretty bleak. The usual approach to a problem is to try and eliminate it. But I just told you that stress cannot and should not be eliminated from your life. It can be the spice of life. So what do you do? Develop a grin-and-bear-it attitude? Hold on and hope for the best? A far better solution is to take a closer look at stress and then learn how to cope with it best.

In reality, stress is something of a neutral element. It is neither good nor bad in itself. What makes stress good or bad is how we handle it. Perhaps two examples might help explain this.

I have a friend who is a salesman. By any standard, his world is filled with pressure. He's in a highly competitive field where only the best survive. And there's no room for mediocrity. The month-end tally becomes the biggest indicator of whether you have made it or not. Even Jack's play is competitive. Put him on a golf course and he plays like Arnold Palmer—for the pin. Get him on a handball court and he's a tiger. He works hard and plays hard. He loves his wife and three kids. He spends time during the week and weekends with them. Jack loves it. He's always on top of things, never sick. A real "energy" type of guy.

On most stress inventories, he would score in the "highly stressed" category. Shoot right off the top. You would suspect such things as fatigue, high blood pressure, perhaps an alcohol problem, ulcers, and heart trouble. Instead, Jack has an unbelievable amount of energy and stamina. Why? For Jack, the challenge of making it as a salesman is just the ingredient that makes life exciting and worthwhile. He made it his spice of life. He successfully turned stress into a positive element.

Now take Norman. Norman has inherited a family business that was an established firm. When he took over he added a subsidiary that allowed him to do his own thing—remodeling. In time, he sold the family business for a good profit, and retained his small company of remodeling.

Today, his working conditions are ideal. He doesn't have to go to work if he doesn't want to. He doesn't have to worry about his income. His home is very comfortable and well appointed. He tells me that his wife and he have a good relationship, sexually and otherwise. His two children are doing well in school. His home is paid for and he's bought a vacation spot on Lake Michigan. He will soon celebrate his twentieth wedding anniversary. He flies his own plane and travels extensively. In short, Norman seems to have it made.

Unfortunately, Norman is a very unhappy man. Despite the fact that he apparently experiences little stress, he complains of chronic fatigue. He has all of the symptoms of high-level stress, yet most stress inventories score him in the "mellow" range. It's Norman's orderly and calm life that is causing the stress. The very lack of change has become a stressful point with him. He's frustrated, hostile, and angry. He wants to do something to prove himself. But he's afraid. Afraid that he'll blow it all financially and his secure environment will be shattered.

Of course, these stories aren't typical, but they illustrate a very important point. It's not stress and change that are doing these people in, it's their attitude toward these things. Jack doesn't have fatigue or lack of energy. He enjoys what he's doing and is coping very well. Norman has troubles—he's not coping properly.

We all have varying degrees of stress. The real question is how well we handle the stress we face. Jack has turned his stress into eustress, or good stress. Norman has let his become distress. And that's where energy enters the picture. Or leaves it.

The Relationship of Stress to Energy

Since we cannot avoid stress, we have two responses available to us. One, we can be governed by stress, and allow it to destroy us. Or we can meet it efficiently, and enjoy it. The first response depletes our supply of energy, the second adds to it. It's almost that simple. Let's take a closer look at how stress can be allowed to rob us of our energy.

In the 1930s, Selye came up with a phrase to describe how stress affects the human body. He called it the general adaptation syndrome, and it merely identifies three responses to stress: alarm, resistance, and exhaustion. The alarm stage is the sense of excitement you get when the boss calls you at home at 7:00 A.M. and asks you to come to work early. Your nervous and endocrine systems move into action. You get a surge of adrenalin that causes an increase in your pulserate and, perhaps, some perspiration under your arms. Blood pressure rises; muscles tense. You're hyped up and ready to go. This response is rather short and often is good for you. For example, if you heard the smoke alarm sound off in the middle of the night, the extra dose of adrenalin your body receives may save your life by allowing you to perform superhuman efforts to get your family to safety. In this stage, stress produces energy to help you complete a task.

If the stress continues, the alarm stage changes to resistance. That is, rather than reacting, your body has decided to fight. The pituitary giand begins producing hormones that equip your body for a longer contest. One hormone, vasopressin, raises your blood pressure, while another, thyrotrophic hormone (TSH), stimulates your thyroid gland, thus accelerating your metabolism. Still another hormone, called adrenocorticotrophic hormone (ACTH), is released, which causes elevated blood sugar levels and alters your immunity system. All of these changes provide you with the sustained energy necessary to keep going.

Under normal circumstances, the second stage gives way to exhaustion, and the body is allowed to rest and recover. This could be characterized by a singularly rough day at the office. You were still in the alarm stage when you got to your desk and found a note from the boss telling you to have a difficult report to him by three o'clock that afternoon. The initial boost of adrenalin gives you the drive to get right at it. Soon you were busy at work trying to make the deadline despite numerous phone interruptions. Things went quite well because the resistance phase was providing the necessary stimulus to your system for you to meet the challenge. When you got home, you were able to relax, read the newspaper, enjoy a nice meal, and get to bed early.

If everyone followed that pattern of adaptation to stress, there would be no need for advice on stress. However, when the stress continues to such an extent that we have no real exhaustion phase, it becomes a very real energy-related problem. Stress at the office, insufficient finances, deteriorating relation-ships, and nagging doubts about your own self-worth result in the following crippling cycle: stress, mental exhaustion, more stress, insomnia, chronic fatigue, more stress, etc.

What many people don't realize about stress is that it produces physical as well as emotional and mental exhaustion. This can easily be demonstrated with the use of an electromyograph (EMG), an instrument that measures the strength of a muscle contraction. When you perform a physical activity such as opening a window, your brain tells the muscles involved how and when to contract so that you can perform the task. This, of course, is done instantly and automatically. These learned patterns of muscle contractions, or engrams, enable you to carry out an infinite number of physical tasks without thinking. Interestingly, even the suggestion of a task will command those muscles to contract. Hence, the sound of the alarm clock in the morning and the subsequent thought of going to work can produce measurable contractions in your muscles, even before you move. Worry over paying the bills or making a speech can cause neck and shoulders muscles to contract. In other words, involuntary mental activity can elicit a physical response. Consequently, you can feel physically tired at the end of a day even though you spent most of your time sitting.

Inborn traits play a crucial role in stress. For example, Selye says that some people are born to be race horses and others to be turtles. If you force a race horse to be a turtle and vice versa, you create significant stress. This is the mistake of the Type A and Type B advocates. Drs. Mayer Friedman and Ray Rosemann from San Francisco have postulated that there are certain people who are more coronary prone. These people are classified as Type A personalities; individuals who try to squeeze 25 hours into 24, who keep taking on more and more responsibilities with less and less time, people who try to do two or more things at a time (such as shaving and driving a car), have a difficult time saying no, are very punctual and competitive, and who do not take time to enjoy their environment. They are the classic workaholics.

At the other end of the spectrum are the Type B's. These individuals take a more relaxed approach to life. They are productive, but they tackle one task at a time, are less impatient, accept themselves, and do take time to stop and smell the roses.

Rosemann and Friedman advocate that people who are Type A should start to adopt more of Type B's behavior characteristics.

Quite frankly, I have problems with the Type A–Type B concept as it is *usually presented*. First, I find it ludicrous to classify four billion people into two distinct categories, A or B. Second, trying to change a supposedly Type A person into a Type B person is stress-producing. If a person likes himself as he is, there is no reason to change. This gets to the concept that Selye mentioned —it's difficult to change a race horse into a turtle and vice versa. Everyone must learn to move at his own pace and by his own rhythms. That is, he must learn to communicate well with his inner feelings. (I will admit, however, that more people who exhibit Type A behaviors want to change than the Type B people.)

Third, the real issue is not Type A versus Type B. It's the traits that Rosemann and Friedman tacked on at the end of their definition—that Type A people are angry, hostile, impatient, aggressive, and that they view life as a struggle. If you have those behavior characteristics, you're in trouble, whether you're Type A or Type B. You're not coping well with your environment. However, I know people who are happy, outgoing, productive, and fun-loving, yet they have Type A characteristics. But they are not hostile. They are not angry. They love life. Life is not a struggle but a joy. Many Type B people are the same way, but I also know some Bs who are very angry, competitive, hostile, and impatient. Life to them is a struggle.

Some stress-management people might argue with me, but I feel the emphasis should be on the devastating attitudes and behaviors associated with anger, impatience, and struggle. These characteristics are an indication that the affected individuals are not coping very well with stress or change in their environment.

Stress need *not* rob you of energy. The key to stress and energy is how you handle it—whether you can manage stress or allow it to manage you. And that's why trying to avoid stress just doesn't work. You can run away from it all, build a log cabin in the wilderness, and sit by the fire the rest of your life and still be plagued by stress—if you are a worrier, uncomfortable with change, and angry at the world. It's all a matter of learning how to cope with stress and understanding your place in the world.

You must remember that stress can be the very element that makes life exciting. It would be impossible to enjoy sex, love, football games, a breath of fresh air, a good book, or music without your hormones that respond to stress. While stress can be debilitating it can also add a tremendous zest to your life. You must find the proper balance between the two. This balance permits a certain amount of stimulation and a certain degree of relaxation. Of course, that sounds easy, but we both know it's not. Yet the information in the third section of the book will help you achieve and maintain that balance of stimulation and relaxation.

CHAPTER 2
Fellowship of the Fatigued

The very word "fatigue" makes me tired. I would just as soon not mention it at all. But you can't talk about energy without dealing with the problem of fatigue. While it is true that our energy level potentials are dictated by heredity, it is apparent that many people are not reaching their optimum level of performance. Fatigue, for whatever reason, is short-circuiting their maximum personal energy.

This country faced an energy shortage long before we realized that we were running out of fossil fuels. Now, many Americans are discovering that even though they pour high-grade fuel into themselves, they still don't run right. Even though they're running miles, doing yoga, going vegetarian, and practicing relaxation, they still are tuckered out, whipped, exhausted, pooped, or burned out. Even though they have focused on "me," the energy they were striving for isn't there. They can't seem to find the necessary energy to perform their duties, live up to their responsibilities, or achieve their goals.

We have lost our zip. We no longer have the drive we had as teenagers or as young adults. Our pattern of living is described best as existing. We awaken, drag ourselves grudgingly to work, return home too tired to do anything but read the paper, then watch TV until we fall asleep. Life has lost its fizz. Even those of us who have the drive and desire to do our jobs well find it practically impossible to return home in the evening full of vim and vigor. The prospect of an evening of dancing, bowling, or some other form of recreation is almost overwhelming.

This phenomenon of fatigue isn't just a product of my imagination. The fatigue of American citizens is frighteningly measurable. The U.S. Government is alarmed by the fact that the productivity of the American worker has declined dramatically. And while it would be naive for me to assume that the loss of productivity is solely dependent upon fatigue (I recognize that the decline in our productivity may be due to a witch's brew of government regulations, foreign competition, OPEC [Organization of Petroleum Exporting Countries], and a loss of the work ethic), there is something to the theory that we physically do not seem to have the energy to do the task at hand.

Many school administrators with whom I work tell me that their biggest staff problem is teacher apathy and burn-out. Fine men and women enter the profession with vitality only to lose their zest for teaching within a few short years. The same can be said in practically every profession. In spite of the fact that we live in a land of plenty where life apparently zooms along at the speed of sound, individually we are victims of fatigue.

To make sure that we are all on the same wavelength, I think it is important to define fatigue. We have all felt it. We say it means exhaustion. That's okay, but we also have experienced different kinds of fatigue.

When you work all day in the garden and collapse in an easy chair at night, is that fatigue? When you feel completely drained of energy after an argument with your boss, is that fatigue? What about that sluggish Monday morning "blah" feeling; is that fatigue?

Fatigue: What Is It?

Fatigue is a confusing term. It means different things to different people. First, let's understand one thing: there's both acute and chronic fatigue. Acute fatigue is easy to identify. A carpenter who has just swung a hammer for eight hours would think something was wrong if his arm wasn't fatigued. Run a marathon some time and see if that doesn't leave you bushed. These are examples of acute fatigue. The cure is simple. All you need is a little rest and relaxation. Acute fatigue responds readily to rest or even simply to switching to another activity. Similarly, a long session of reading, studying, or other intense mental concentration may leave your brain spent, and can be cured by simply giving it a break—with rest or some physical activity. Dr. Hans Selye, who I introduced to you in Chapter 1, has noted that "a voluntary change of activity is as good or even better than rest . . . For example, when either fatigue or forced interruption prevents us from finishing a mathematical problem, it is better to go for a swim than simply sit around. Substituting demands on our musculature for those previously made on the intellect not only gives our brain a rest but helps us avoid worrying about the frustrating interruption. Stress on one system helps to relax another."

In this book I'm not concerned about this type of fatigue. It is easily recognized and readily cured. Furthermore, acute fatigue represents no long-term drain on your personal energy reserves. In fact, I view them as good symptoms, evidence that you are already performing at high energy levels, needing only occasional recuperation breaks.

It's another type of fatigue—chronic fatigue—that concerns me. Those who suffer from chronic fatigue don't get tired once in a while. They stay tired, week after week, month after month, year after year. The fatigue does not seem to respond to rest, recreation, or medication. And, occasionally, when it does subside it returns in a matter of days or weeks.

A thorough physical examination by your physician usually reveals nothing. But the patient complains, and his or her feelings are very real. "I don't have the energy I once had. Things are a drag."

It's been estimated that half of the people who go to see their family physician have nothing organically wrong with them, just overwhelming fatigue or a feeling that they lack energy.

Chronic fatigue, simply stated, is a pervasive feeling of a total shortage of energy. If you're able to function at all, it is only due to an immense effort of the will. You feel as though the force of gravity has doubled when it comes to getting out of bed in the morning. Relationships seem to require more effort than they're worth. Your job is like a dead weight. You wonder why you've stayed with it so long. Your very shoes seem to have rubber cement gumming up their soles, holding you back. A tremendous amount of willpower must be mustered to do anything out of the daily routine of things. And even the daily routine can get to be too much. How many times have you thought, "I'm too tired to get off the couch and crawl into bed." When there's no energy for picking up after yourself or brushing your teeth, and you want to switch channels on the TV but can't get up, that's chronic fatigue.

People who suffer from this type of chronic fatigue cut across all socio-economic lines. They include corporate ladder climbers, decision-makers, custodians, teachers, ministers, housewives, truck drivers, doctors, students, and so forth. Ofttimes they are individuals who have had their nose to the grindstone for 20 years or more. Now they find themselves physically and emotionally bankrupt. Their brain seems to have wilted and all body functions have gone limp with it.

I've also known high school and college students who are chronically tired.

Individuals who claim that they are too tired to take up running, go backpacking, or take a course overload. As I'm writing this chapter, I'm returning from a workshop that involved 300 young elementary school teachers, between the ages of 21 and 35. Their complaint was burn-out and chronic fatigue. The energy level of the group was abysmally low.

As you have surmised, chronic fatigue may be caused by things inside and outside of your being. Those from within include such things as poor nutrition, illness, and lack of fitness. Those from without are poor relationships and the stress or strain of living. You may also have guessed that there is a very close relationship between the two.

Chronic fatigue can attack both your physical and psychological being. Scientists tell us that like acute fatigue, there are three types of chronic fatigue: physical, mental, and emotional. These three are so closely intertwined that it is impossible to separate them. But to help you better understand them, I'm separating them here so that you can see their influence on your energy levels. Remember, though, that they are closely related. Physical fatigue can cause emotional fatigue, emotional fatigue can cause mental fatigue, and mental fatigue can drain you both physically and emotionally.

Physical Fatigue

Physical fatigue may have physiological or pathological causes. The physiological fatigue includes such things as weariness that occurs from a lack of fitness. Your level of physical fitness dictates when your daily physical fatigue will occur and how long you will be able to hold it off. Regardless, the fatigue will come. For example, a fit person may be able to do his daily chores and then go out for an evening of partying, dancing, or socializing. The unfit person, on the other hand, may be exhausted by two or three in the afternoon, and find the idea of taking a walk in the evening impossible.

Pathological fatigue, on the other hand, includes fatigue due to high blood pressure, diabetes, obesity, hypoglycemia, and arteriosclerosis. In other words, fatigue caused by some disease state. I have a good friend, Dave, who suffers from high blood pressure that is hereditary. He is whipped by four o'clock in the afternoon. When he wakes up he feels good, but as the day wears on his blood pressure starts to wear him down. His ability to function is markedly impaired. He wants to leave the office. He says he's a paper shuffler by this time and simply sits there counting the four walls until quitting time. His fatigue comes not from a lack of fitness, but from a disease state.

As you might surmise, physiological and pathological fatigue can go hand in hand. Many times people who improve their fitness level find that their blood pressure drops or some other ailment disappears. So there's a very close inter-play between pathological and physiological fatigue.

Mental Fatigue

Mental fatigue is synonymous with boredom. Yawning, sleepiness, and drowsiness are the usual characteristics. Mental fatigue frequently occurs when you do the same task over and over again. Many writers suffer from mental fatigue after a book is completed. They have taxed their thinking and creative processes to the limit. Many students at the end of the school year are also exhausted mentally.

Generally, though not always, rest, sleep, an improvement of physical fitness or nutrition will help solve physical and chronic mental fatigue.

Emotional Fatigue

Emotional fatigue is radically different from physical and mental fatigue. Its causes are insidious. Its cure is complex. Emotional fatigue is usually associated with hurrying, worrying, emotional stress, a fast-paced society, working against the clock, struggling against ill-defined goals, obstacles that seem insurmountable, and change.

Mental fatigue seems to be relieved by rest and a change of some physical condition. Physical fatigue is relieved by rest and proper physical fitness. Emotional fatigue is another story. The worried executive who tries to sleep his problems away only finds that he sleeps fitfully. And then, when he wakes up, he still feels exhausted. As he dreams he feels he's frustrated, unable to get away from the bear on his back. He dreams one frustrating situation after another. He runs from the enemy but his legs won't move. Conflicts are unresolved. Goals are not achieved.

Eighty percent or more of the chronic fatigue problems that people experience are due to emotional fatigue. After a period of time the real and dreamed worries, the hyped-up environment, and the radical changes that have taken place in one's life create problems such as boredom, anger, depression, and anxiety. These in turn destroy energy levels.

Boredom

Many times boredom produces mental fatigue; but it can also be a precipitator of chronic emotional fatigue. In industrialized America many jobs are monotonous. Putting the 32nd bolt on a car in an assembly line is a perfect example. But even supposedly technical jobs can be boring. Personally, if I have to conduct one more exercise stress test I'm going to scream. Physicians have told me that they are bored with the routine of their medical practice: examination after examination after examination.

The problem here is sameness, a day-in-and-day-out routine that can cause a lack of stimulation to the brain, nervous and hormonal systems. Extra hormones are not secreted, so we are extremely sleepy and lethargic. That is, unless something out of the ordinary happens. The assembly-line worker becomes alert if the assembly line speeds up. Things can change for me if Bruce Jenner walks into my stress-testing lab. And a doctor involved in a life and death struggle to save his heart-fibrillating patient will not be bored. When these things happen, our approach to our job changes dramatically and we feel full of vim and vigor.

One of the biggest problems with boredom is that bored people tend to shut off their emotions. They become numb to the world. This numbing phenomenon reduces your feelings of energy for both physiological and psychological reasons. Psychologically it occurs because we want to survive the tedium of the job. Physiologically it may be due to the fact that your brain may secrete selected hormones that turn down your brain's perceptions.

Depression

If you're caught in a state of depression or despondency, you probably also have low levels of energy. Unfortunately, feelings of lost energy tend to feed upon themselves in a vicious, unrelenting circle. When feeling depressed you experience inertia. You don't want to do anything—physically, mentally, or emotionally. You're not satisfied with the way you're handling life's problems. You become even more depressed. The more depressed you are the more you try to escape reality with sleep. More sleep produces less physical activity and less physical activity produces even lower energy levels. These lessened energy levels produce even more depression and soon you're centering on a depressed or decreased self-concept.

The poor self-concept can cause even lower and lower levels of energy and turn you more and more inward. Your behavior becomes erratic and you soon experience total inertia—a point at which you just can't seem to get anything together. Psychologist Dr. Wayne Dyer, in his book *The Sky's the Limit*, describes inertia thus:

> A state of being in which you are unable to move yourself, incapable of action. In this state you will be either motionless or carried along "the way you were going before" or the way others direct or push you. In terms of problem-solving, inertia often follows

a spasm of panic. Emotionally it is usually associated with depression and/or boredom. If depression is chronic indeed, or the boredom is "existentialist"—that is, it is not boredom with this or that situation or activity, but with life—it can lead to psychosis and/or suicide. . . . Depression and boredom result in a lack of initiative about everything, in passive behavior such as staying in bed or at home doing nothing but feeling sorry for yourself.

Emotionally drained, you feel depressed. Your self-concept isn't very good either. The depression becomes deeper and the "slow-down" part of your nervous system may become activated. General fatigue sets in. You have very little energy, if any. Soon you start to experience anger. Because your self-concept isn't what it should be, you repress it.

Anger

Anger is another energy problem. Anger stimulates your nervous system. Blood pressure rises, heart rate increases, and hormones are secreted. You explode!

The venting of your spleen in anger offers good news and bad news. The good news is that you probably dissipate your emotions and relax your muscle tension. The bad news is that the recipient of your outburst may lash back at you, only serving to heighten your anger and create a greater sympathetic response on your part. While arguing you may be full of energy, but afterwards you feel whipped because of the tremendous emotional-physical strain placed on your body.

A second part of the bad news may be that the recipient of your outburst is hurt, producing feelings of guilt on your part that only add to your stress.

Repression of your anger doesn't work here either. Anger stimulates your nervous system, but when you repress your anger you create a strange set of affairs. Let's say you and your spouse have a difference of opinion. You decide to keep your feelings inside. After all, you've been taught since childhood that it's not nice to get mad—to show your emotions. So you throttle your feelings. Anger excites your nervous system and activates secretion of hormones. They start to predominate as you get angrier and angrier. You're getting ready for your body to act. You repress your outburst, however. Your muscles are tense, your blood pressure is high, sugar is secreted, and extra hormones are circulating in your bloodstream. You're fighting like mad to keep the emotions inside. Suddenly you feel tired. Emotionally drained. You retire to bed or to sleep. You toss and turn. Sleep finally comes. But it's not truly restful. You awaken exhausted. Your nervous system again wants to act, but you put a damper on it. You're still angry but you don't do anything about it. Now you become depressed. You're upset with your pettiness. You do devious, subtle things to get back at your spouse, or you become a doormat—saying "yes dear," "no dear." The latter occurs because you are ashamed of your anger and pettiness.

The body interprets all of this and uses its protective mechanism of depression to help you handle your angry feelings. You have felt so much stimulation, so much anger, and so much hostility, that the only way you can protect your body is by shutting down. The result is an extremely low level of energy. But you don't read it as that. You read it as an inability to control your life and feelings.

Slowly your self-concept slips, and more depression occurs. The deeper the depression, the more inertia. Soon a vicious cycle of anger, depression, inertia, poor-self-concept, back to anger is set up. And you don't give a damn about anything.

Of course, other emotions such as guilt and jealousy are also kept inside and probably produce a similar response to anger. In fact, the guilt and jealousy probably cause you to be angrier still, and the same cycle starts again.

Anxiety

While depression or anger can cause feelings of lack of energy, so can anxiety. Anxiety is closely allied with depression. In fact psychologists say there is a continuum with depression at one end and anxiety at the other. Ofttimes, a person is anxious first and as the anxiety builds and heightens it progresses into depression. Depression, quite frankly, is the circuit breaker for anxiety. Anxiety-producing situations cause people to get more and more whipped up. They keep taking on more and more input of fear, anticipation of something stressful, and worry. They become more and more apprehensive. Soon the anxiety interferes with their ability to concentrate. That is followed by psychosomatic symptoms which produce more anxiety. Hormone levels skyrocket. The body rebels and starts to shut down. Depression follows. They then become anxious about depression.

The anxiety, depression, and back to anxiety circle occurs simply because they have disrupted the internal balance of their hormonal and nervous systems. Soon their body is caught in an overload. To protect the body, the various systems shut down and they become depressed. The result is less and less energy.

Emotional fatigue causes a sensory overload. It takes your mind, body, and emotions beyond your ability to cope. Research done by the National Institute of Mental Health illustrates this point. Experiments with an electroencephalo-gram indicate that the brain controls a "sensoristat" that helps us control the effects of sensory stimulation. When you are overstimulated emotionally, this mechanism dials down to prevent an overload. If you are exposed to high levels of pressure, responsibility, and change, the sensoristat dims your perception to protect you. And that response results in feelings of lethargy and fatigue. Often, such an overload brings about total collapse. More often, however, it creates that frustrating feeling of not having enough steam to get through the day.

CHAPTER 3
An Old Body in a Brave New World

Winter was coming, and Fred the caveman began to prepare for the cold weather. He sharpened his flint axe and hiked off into the woods to fell a mighty tree. As he whittled away at the tree, his strenuous labor was interrupted by a roar and a growl that struck fear in his heart. Sure enough, a large and angry prehistoric beast was closing in on him. Without even thinking, he heaved his mighty axe at the beast, which bounced off its rough hide, angering the creature even more. Not particularly wanting to become a midday snack for the menacing predator, Fred did what any self-respecting Cro-Magnon would do when faced with danger: he ran. Lickety-split, out of the woods, over the meadow, up the side of the mountain, and into his cave. He shoved the stone across the opening, and the unlucky beast went without lunch. Fred's heart was pounding, his chest was heaving. But he was safe. He poured a tall glass of guava juice, put his feet up on a rock, and settled in for a nice, relaxing nap.

This fanciful scenario illustrates that for years humans were involved in a life-and-death struggle with their environment. Their minds and bodies were well equipped for survival. Their strong and fit bodies gave them the capability to survive stressful situations. They were outfitted with a psychological and physiological make-up that permitted them to run long or fight hard if attacked or challenged.

In many ways, we are a lot like early man. When he was attacked by an animal or another human his nerves and glands would make necessary adjustments to improve his chances for survival. The grey matter of his brain told him that danger was imminent and signaled the hypothalamus—that small, specialized tissue that is the key to many of man's bodily adjustments. The

19

hypothalamus, in turn, relayed the same message to the nervous and endocrine systems. The key centers activated were the sympathetic nervous system (the stimulating part of your autonomic nervous system of your body), and the pituitary gland.

The sympathetic nervous system stimulated the liver, which increased the blood's clotting capacity so that if early man were cut in battle he would be less likely to bleed to death. The fat stored on his body was mobilized so that it could be used for energy in a lengthy fight or to help him run as fast and as far away as possible.

The heart rate was speeded up to provide additional oxygen to the muscles and to carry away energy-robbing carbon dioxide. Muscle tension was increased and extra blood sent to the muscles so that man could respond physically, and then the hormones began to flow.

The pituitary gland was also activated and gave off hormones that activated the adrenals and the liver. These glands then secreted their own hormones.

The pancreas was also stimulated and insulin production was increased. Release of these hormones in turn caused an increase in blood fats and sugars so that the activity could be maintained for a longer period of time.

These carefully orchestrated physiological changes caused and permitted man to spring into action. He fought or ran long and hard to survive. As he did, the extra secreted hormones and the nervous tension of the muscles were utilized, as were his blood fats and sugars. At the conclusion of the battle there was a tremendous physical letdown. In fact, he may have been forced to stop or slow down during the battle because of extreme physical fatigue. Regardless, when the event was over he was bushed. His parasympathetic nervous system (the calming part of his autonomic nervous system) took over and he was ready for some rest and sleep as his body wound down. It is only conjecture on my part but I'm sure he felt a good bit of satisfaction regarding the day's event. Though fatigued and physically exhausted, he had met the enemy and won. I'm sure such a feeling was ego-building. He felt like tomorrow was going to be another day and that he was ready for its challenges, experiences, and victories. Life back then was simple. The enemy was well known—other humans, animals, and the hostile environment.

Today, our bodies have inherited the same mechanisms. When we are faced with stress our hypothalamus is stimulated and our sympathetic nervous system and hormones swing into action. But instead of saber-toothed tigers and invading barbarians, we are confronted by crowds, job frustrations, domestic responsibilities, social demands, and change. Although these challenges are mental in nature, our brain perceives them as dangerous. The message it sends to the body is the same one Fred received: fight or flight.

Unfortunately, our response today is short-circuited. First, we don't know who or where the enemy is. Second, we have many potential stresses hitting us at one time. Third, we don't know how to respond to our enemies, or we have been chastised since childhood to keep things inside. So we adopt a martyr's attitude. We internalize our frustrations, anxieties, and hostility. It is not socially acceptable to run away from the office or to punch the ulcer-producing boss in the nose when we fail to meet his standards. Instead, we passively sit and take it. The very idea of sitting on our feelings and not doing something physical is counter to our heritage. Immobilization in attitude and action causes significant problems because first, we are not fit enough to handle the pressure, and secondly, the sitting produces a nervous and endocrine response that is not dissipated as it should be.

In earlier times, man lived by his strength and endurance almost alone. Every one of his daily tasks required the vigorous and dynamic use of his body. Success in life meant being able to run fast and long and to strike hard if attacked. Fitness was necessary for survival. As man progressed, so did his mind. He started to use tools and animals, and his work became a little easier. Still, man's brawn had to be used if he was to survive.

Then suddenly a dramatic change occurred. The Industrial Revolution brought with it a way of life totally alien to man. The automobile became king. People moved to suburbia, shopping centers sprang up, interstate highways connected cities, and walking was abandoned. Ranch homes became the rule and fewer two-story homes were built.

Today, actual physical labor is almost nonexistent. Gardens and yards are often now maintained by power mowers, tillers, and cultivators. Leaves are scooped up in power-driven vacuum cleaners. The house is heated by gas or oil —no more chopping wood and shoveling coal. Clothing is washed in automatic washers, and dried in dryers. There is no more hand scrubbing and hanging on a line to dry. Rugs are vacuumed, turning the annual spring ritual of beating the carpets into a museum showpiece. The list is endless and frightening when you realize that deep inside of each of us is a mechanism that is screaming, "Run, throw, jump, pull, duck, fight, swim!" Modern technology has created a lifestyle in which the great majority of people in industrialized societies do not have to do much physical work—at home or on the job. So our fitness slips; our fitness to fight or our fitness to handle stress.

Interestingly, this problem is not seen in primitive societies, where threats to life and security are more often in physical forms that demand direct, physical responses. Threatened by hunger, thirst, natural phenomena, or living enemies, the people in nontechnological societies act naturally to avert the threat, and the action discharges the stored energy before it has a chance to accumulate and cause severe emotional fatigue. The primitive may be tired physically, but he does not have physical fatigue due to emotional wipeout.

One frightening experience (a near accident), an argument with the boss, or a disappointing performance will not insult your body. You are a lot tougher than that! But the constant pressure of a bad marriage, a poor relationship with your children, a hated job, and a list of other conflicts can and will cause the body (particularly the sympathetic nervous and endocrine systems) to be over-worked, and cause overstimulation. This overstimulation manifests itself first with physical, mental, and especially emotional fatigue.

Fred had an option that most of us don't take advantage of. He was a physical person. That helped him cope. As much as we don't like to admit it, we are no longer physical people, regardless of the occurrence of what has been called a fitness boom. Despite the fact that many Americans picture themselves as active, most are not. Scientists have been able to demonstrate that. They've been able to show that the fitness levels of North Americans have declined. They also know that once a basic level of fitness is lost, there is little you can do to fight stress and to have the energy to survive unless you rebuild your fitness level.

Research on Fitness

Let me show you some of the research documentation that shows that North Americans are fatigued because of a lack of fitness. Dr. Donald Bailey, a professor at the University of Saskatchewan in Western Canada, along with Dr. Roy Shephard of the University of Toronto, tested 672 women and 558 men to find out their fitness levels. The results indicated that these Canadian men and women, measured for their fitness levels, tested poorly. And the women were somewhat worse than the men. The least fit group of all were young women in their 20s.

Over half the women aged 20 to 29 were well below the average fitness level for their age group. Forty-six percent of the women in their 30s also scored below average.

There's no reason to expect that the U.S. citizens would fare any better. In fact, small studies done at various locations in the United States suggest that we may be less fit.

A primary reason for the decline in fitness levels is that while we are active socially, politically, and domestically, we are not active physically. Look at these facts: Back in the 1930s, the average American male expended 3,000 calories a day. The average female expended 2,400. Today, the average American male burns off 2,200 calories a day and the average female 1,500. That means that 800 to 900 calories of activity have been programmed out of our lives. Eight hundred to 900 calories is equivalent to an eight- or nine-mile jog per day. The bottom line is, of course, that we do not work *physically* as hard as our predecessors. The result is overwhelming fatigue. We are too tired to get through the day because we have not built up an energy reserve.

What do I mean by energy reserve? The easiest way to describe this is to think of an athlete. When an athlete gets "into shape" he conditions and hardens his body for almost any athletic emergency. That is, if he is expected to put on a sprint at the end of a contest he trains himself so he will be able to do it (and win). To get this reserve he must push himself harder and harder each day. In fact, he must push himself to the point where he will work harder now than he ever will in the athletic event. This gives him that competitive edge.

Not surprisingly, it's the same way with life. If you do the same thing every day, you might be able to "slip through" without any cause for concern. But if you are called upon to do anything extra (like taking a few extra flights of stairs, going out bowling, or fixing a flat tire), your body can't handle it. And in the evening you're pooped. You must condition yourself for that reserve. Improving your fitness level gives you the edge you need to prevent an unexpected letdown and still have the energy for other activities later on in the day. The teachers and professors in my workshops who are unfit can't cope with anything extra. They can't cope with the extra exercise, lectures, and time devoted to the class. It is due to a lack of fitness. The little extra work I ask them to do exhausts them. How do I know? Many tell me that after they're back in shape their stamina for extra activities increases dramatically.

It is a simple fact that the American way of life begets fatigue and a feeling of no energy, and one of the biggest problems is a lack of physical fitness. Despite all the hoopla and attention focused on fitness in this country, the number of Americans who exercise on a regular basis is low.

Most experts agree that regular exercise is participation in any activity for at least three times a week. Work by the President's Council on Physical Fitness and Sports has shown that a large percentage of our adult population does not exercise sufficiently. Most people who do exercise participate only two days a week or less. In fact, 90 percent of the bowlers and tennis players, 83 percent of the golfers, 70 percent of the swimmers, 60 percent of the bicyclists,

50 percent of the joggers, 33 percent of the weight lifters, 30 percent of the walkers, and 23 percent of the people who do calisthenics "do their thing" less frequently than three times a week.

The President's Council has indicated that only 30 million Americans exercise regularly, about 20 percent of our population. Furthermore, they have stated that 45 percent of the population gets no exercise at all!

Other experts see the situation as being even more dismal. Some believe that statistics on the Canadian population are probably closer to the truth about Americans. According to a recent study, only 20 percent of the Canadian population engages in some form of physical activity such as walking for pleasure, jogging, hiking, or other exercise.

Dr. Kenneth Cooper, of *Aerobics* fame, is convinced that the President's Council's estimate that 30 million Americans exercise regularly is an enormous exaggeration. "It's probably more like 10 to 15 million—probably less . . . and even those people aren't exercising regularly."

Exercise physiologist Dr. Paul Lessick is even more pessimistic. He doesn't accept the President's Council estimate that 55 percent of Americans engage in at least some exercise. Applying his own demanding standards, Lessick concludes that only 5 to 7 percent of the population surveyed by the Council perform the proper kind and amount of exercise.

Dr. Elsworth R. Buskirk, director of the Noll Laboratory for Human Performance Research at Pennsylvania State University, concurs. He estimates that less than 5 percent of the present general population exercises regularly.

The most skeptical of all, however, is Dr. Joseph Ahrens, a cardiologist specializing in preventive medicine. He states that "past the age of 35 less than 2 percent of American males and less than 1 percent of American females are physically fit." In other words, only 1 to 2 percent of those people past the age of 35 are getting adequate exercise.

You can take your own poll. Count 100 people on your street who exercise for 15 to 20 minutes three or more times a week throughout the year. See what kind of percentage you get. I did. I live in a small Midwest town. With athletic children included I calculate that 12 percent of the people on my street fulfilled that three-day requirement.

The phenomenon of lack of physical activity is shown in the incidence of obesity. Obesity is rapidly increasing. Of at least 10 million teenagers, 2 out of 10 are too fat. Among adults, 3 out of 10 men and 4 out of 10 women over 40 are more than 20 percent above their ideal weight. Seat manufacturers tell us that they had to design broader-bottomed chairs for our broader-bottomed citizens of the 1980s. Clothing manufacturers report that individuals of both sexes and all ages have shown an increase in appearance of arm, chest, and body measurements.

Not only are we fat, we seem to be getting fatter. A weight gain of a pound each year after age 25 is considered "normal" by most physicians. That means a 150-pound, 25-year-old person can expect to weight 190 pounds by the time he retires. It's little wonder the retiree is characterized as a paunchy, plump, white-haired gnome who is too tired to chew anything but oatmeal, or play anything but dominoes. The good things he never had time for—playing with the kids, outdoor sports, dancing, sex—are now out of his feeble, flabby reach.

Additionally, some experts feel that the food we eat, the very stuff that's supposed to provide us with energy, is a major energy-robber and a significant contributor to the fatigue problem. While our ancestors certainly had nutritional problems connected with the obtaining and preservation of good, wholesome foods, they also had remarkable wisdom in knowing what to eat in order to stay healthy. Largely due to their slower-paced lifestyle, they could take the time to eat properly.

Today, the one criteria for judging a meal seems to be speed: Food is evaluated on whether it can be prepared in a short period of time. If it can be done in 15 minutes or less, that's good. If it takes time, that's bad. Unfortunately, speed comes in boxes, cans, and metal trays—more salt, sugar, and fat, and not much in the way of vitamins, minerals, and complex carbohydrates. The fast-food franchises are involved in a race to put a "take out" on each corner of every intersection in the United States. Even quality restaurants, in an effort to keep prices down, are turning to convenience foods. For example, when was the last time you had real mashed potatoes at a restaurant, not something out of a box? If you think eating out is a casual experience, just remember that it's been estimated that ¼ to ⅓ of all meals eaten are eaten outside of the home—a place where you are rarely given the opportunity to "have it your way." Your way should be minus salt, sugar, saturated fat, and a host of mind-puzzling additives before it comes to your table. Where is the chef that lets you decide how much of these ingredients are best for you?

At the same time, many food processors have shifted the emphasis to heat-and-serve meals that are prefrozen, prepackaged, and ready to pop in the oven 15 minutes before supper time. Some food technicians spend more time devising food that can be eaten without silverware than food that is healthy. The result: instead of wholesome, nutritious foods to fuel our energy demands, too often we eat deep-fried, grease-laden, vitamin- and mineral-deficient, heavily processed food as the main course in our meals.

Prudent food manufacturers know they must give the public a product it wants. The public has demonstrated the desire for foods that are cheap, easy to prepare, and easier to eat. A simple illustration is the potato. Give most people a choice and they'll ask for french fries over baked. The reason? "I can eat it with my fingers." "I don't have time to prepare a baked potato." "I can take 'em right out of a bag and pop them in the oven." "French fries taste better." Yet, by the time a serving of french fries has been thawed from a long term in the freezer, been boiled in a vat of grease, and then sprinkled with more salt than a human needs in a week, the potato has gained over 100 calories, lost a good bit of its nutrition, and picked up two additives of questionable value: grease and salt.

Contributing to this nutrition problem is the absence of fresh foods from our diets. Since our lifestyle does not allow for daily shopping at a fresh-food market, we rely greatly on canned or frozen foods. Consequently, we end up eating some fiber (which is good) but very little nutrition. For example, canned peas lose 38 percent of their vitamins in the canning process and 27 percent in the freezing process. By the time you eat a frozen dinner it has lost 40 percent of the vitamin A, 100 percent of the vitamin C, 80 percent of the B complex vitamins, and 55 percent of the vitamin E. It's like pouring low-octane gasoline into the fuel tank of a high-performance automobile. The engine just doesn't have the pep because the fuel is deficient.

Probably the biggest culprit in the nutrition scam is sugar. In Queen Victoria's time, sugar was a rare luxury that only the wealthy could afford. The fair Queen herself, though they were cleverly hidden by portrait artists, had black teeth from an irrepressible desire for sugar that only she could afford. Now, however, times have changed. Sugar is everywhere. If you don't believe me, grab any food item packaged in a box. Sugar is almost always listed either first or second in the ingredients, which are listed by weight. Such sneak attacks of sugar on the American diet have resulted in an annual consumption of 120 pounds of sugar per person. To put that into perspective, imagine 25 five-pound bags of granulated white sugar sitting there on your food shelves.

What's so bad about sugar? I'll discuss that more in Chapter 12, but briefly, sugar has been implicated in disease conditions that cause some people to have a drastic loss of energy. Many people who experience the feeling of being run down, run out, or run over have a sugar metabolism problem, a condition which falls into a category that could be described as "the slows."

When it comes to surviving in this brave new world of ours we are clobbered. First, we are caught in the midst of a rapidly changing world that stresses us with fast-paced living, changing values, and ill-defined roles. Second, most of us are not fit enough to survive in this world. We are sedentary and eat foods which do us in energy-wise. Years ago, only the fittest survived the onslaughts of nature. Today, only the fittest can make it through this maze of future shock. If you want to enjoy this life to its fullest, if you want to maximize your personal energy, if you want the true pleasure of living at the capacity that is optimal for you, you must take charge and become fit.

Still, many people refuse to believe it. They know their energy is slipping. They know that they don't feel up to par. So people start looking for solutions. But they keep looking for a magic bullet, the one thing that will give them that elusive lift. But, as we shall see in the next chapter, they select aids that defeat them and that take them down a wrong-way street. That is, many people select things that provide temporary lifts but then, eventually they're let down by them.

Perhaps paraphrasing the lines from a 1980 hit song characterizes best the effects of the short-term energy shots; they lift you up, up, up, only to drop you down hard in the long run.

CHAPTER 4
We'll Do Anything for a Rush

Some of the very things people use to obtain energy become negative, energy-reducing addictions. We have become a society that looks to everyone and everything else for the solution to our energy problem, so much so that we have forfeited our freedom to choose the way we live. We smoke, even though we know it's not good for us. We consume too much alcohol, even though it strains relationships, decreases productivity, and reduces personal effectiveness. We use drugs—over-the-counter, prescription, and illegal substances—even though the potential for irreparable harm is frightening. Even our sources of entertainment have become an inescapable trap. No one in his right mind really wants to see another human being maimed and crippled, yet we sit glued to the replays of a cornerback smashing into a wide receiver's neck in a professional football game or flock to hockey arenas that promise 60 minutes of action in the form of bench-clearing brawls.

What is it that compels us to become hooked on these self-destructive preoccupations? It would probably take a roomful of psychiatrists to come up with a thorough answer, but it is my belief that part of the problem lies in our endless search for stimulation. We want a rush—a lift—to help us through the day. We'll do just about anything to get a surge of adrenalin. And often, the things we do are at best energy-robbing, and are often life-threatening.

Smoking

Take smoking, for example. Tobacco addiction in America dates back to
the Indians who were puffing and sniffing dried leaves from the tobacco plant

when Columbus arrived. Early settlers liked the brief lift they got when they passed around the ceremonial peace pipe and they decided that smoking was pretty neat. It soon became not only a source of income for the Middle Atlantic and Southern colonies, it became a way of life for a majority of the adult males. Women came out of the closet in the early twentieth century, and now there are an estimated 65 million smokers in America.

Of course, if smoking was in the same ball park as taking vitamins or grabbing a handful of peanuts occasionally, no one would be worried. But we *are* worried. By the 1940s doctors began to notice an alarming increase in deaths due to lung cancer. Without a great deal of research they were able to correlate this increase with cigarette smoking. Later, they found an association between smoking and many other diseases such as heart disease and bladder cancer. Currently, the dangers of smoking are printed on every pack and the government has conducted a media blitz that condemns the use of cigarettes. We have been given every reason to avoid cigarettes, yet people continue to smoke. Why?

It starts with peer pressure. While boys no longer go behind the barn to sneak a few puffs, most people get started as youngsters, who succumb to the need to be accepted by their friends who think that smoking is the adult thing to do. Soon, however, they find that they *need* to smoke. They need that little lift to get them started in the morning. They are hooked because they need the stimulus a cigarette provides, to get going, to relax. Ask a person why he lights up first thing in the morning and he'll say, "It wakes me up." Ask him why he smokes after supper and he'll say, "It relaxes me." As incongruous as it may seem, some people have become convinced that the only way to get a lift or to mellow out is to smoke. And, interestingly, smoking seems to do both.

First, the nicotine in smoke reacts with the acetylcholine receptors of the brain. Acetylcholine is a nerve transmitter in the brain. This interaction causes the autonomic nervous system to respond. The nicotine causes extra adrenalin to be secreted. As a result, there's an increase in blood pressure, heart rate, cardiac output, and blood sugar level. In other words, a smoker gets a rush, a surge of energy, albeit nervous energy. He's hyped up and ready to go.

Shortly after that initial lift, however, the body tends to slow down. And that explains how cigarettes can have a calming effect. In essence, the smoker is strangling himself. The gases he absorbs restrict his circulation. Any time a person inhales smoke he's ingesting carbon monoxide. In addition to being toxic, carbon monoxide prevents smokers from getting the usual amount of life-giving oxygen. The general slowing-down effect of smoking is really a subtle energy drain, hence a sense of relaxation. Instead of actually calming down and relaxing, a smoker is merely pulling the plug on his energy supply. Repeated smoking adds to this depletion of energy. Usually smokers smoke one to three cigarettes an hour. Just as the body starts to slow down, the smoker feels he needs a lift. One puff and he stimulates his body again. But soon the body must rest and fatigue sets in. As a result, when a smoker lights up to fight fatigue he's really beating a dead horse. And, if you're the smoker, the dead horse is yourself.

To the addicted smoker, that explanation doesn't matter a bit. He feels that lift in the morning and he feels that calming effect after supper. He has convinced himself that his habit is the best way to stimulate whatever it is that produces those desirable effects. He is also willing to put up with minor throat irritations, unnecessary coughing, decreased sex drive and response, premature wrinkling of skin, as well as the very real threat of heart disease and cancer.

Reinforcing the smoker's dependency on tobacco are the nasty things that happen to him when he tries to quit. He becomes extremely jittery. Little things upset him. He is irritable. All of these problems convince him that he needs to resume his habit in order to get back in control. What has happened is that he has lost his security blanket—his crutch. Eventually, he can take it no longer. He needs that stimulation that smoking provides. He starts smoking again.

Alcohol

But smoking isn't enough. In man's quest for more and more stimulation he turns to alcohol. Initially, there is nothing more stimulating than a couple of drinks. Have a few beers at the ball park and you will cheer louder and laugh more than the teetotaler. Have a couple of cocktails instead of lunch and you will impress everyone with your witty and urbane conversation. We have convinced ourselves that everything from hobbies to parties are more enjoyable with a can or glass in one of our hands.

The problem with this line of thinking is that alcohol's lift is promptly followed by a depressing slow-down of a person's entire system. In fact, alcohol is classified by the medical profession not as a stimulant, but as a depressant. The initial surge of energy you get from a drink or two is rather short lived. In a short period of time you're going to feel tired and irritable. If you were in the proper setting, you would probably fall asleep for an energy-building catnap. Unfortunately, most people drink in settings that do not allow a nap —during lunch hour, at a bar that's a 20-minute drive from home, at a party in another part of town. By the way, the tired feeling many people experience after a drink or two may be due to a sludging of the blood cells. Hence, less energy-giving oxygen is carried to the body's cells—especially the brain cells. The end product is fatigue.

A lot of people like to make the distinction between social drinking and problem drinking. I recognize that an occasional drink or two is not going to pose a serious energy problem. Drinking for some people may not be harmful at all. In moderation (no more than one or two drinks per day) alcohol may lower their blood pressure and act as a mild and fairly safe sedative. It may even help some people to relax, socialize, and enjoy their meals better. Yet I think these people are a minority. The increase in alcoholism and alcohol-related problems indicates that many people are drinking for all of the wrong reasons. Even the idea that alcohol is relaxing may be misleading. Certain properties in alcohol have qualities similar to morphine—which means that alcohol can act as a sedative. Also, don't forget the sludging of cells. Unfortunately, long-time alcohol misuse can destroy energy. There is evidence that the heart muscle may undergo a type of degeneration in regular alcohol-users, while at the same time, brain cells and liver tissue may also be destroyed. These changes will induce fatigue in the long run. Despite all of this, people insist that alcohol revs 'em up—gets them going.

The Pill Generation

Never before have Americans of all ages consumed so many sleeping pills, pep pills, diet pills, sedatives, and tranquilizers. We have pills—both prescribed and over-the-counter—for every purpose and many with no real purpose at all. People, with the help of media advertising and their friendly physicians, have discovered the easy way out of their problem. They have been convinced that there is nothing that can't be cured by the right pharmaceutical concoction.

There are some people who take a pill every morning to clear the cobwebs, and every evening take another pill to help them sleep. Still others take pills to lose weight or pills to reduce anxiety. Drugs have become a way of life. We turn to them for assistance instead of learning to handle our problems in a mature, self-reliant manner.

Amphetamines are used by millions of Americans for stimulation. Speed hypes you up with nervous energy for a very concrete reason. It increases the activity of some of your hormones that heighten brain activity and make you so jittery that most users cannot sit still. Not satisfied with the amphetamine hype, cocaine is being used. Coke is the quick-energy drug preferred by musicians and entertainers. Its use is increasing each year in professional basketball, for example, to the point that at least one National Basketball Association (NBA) official claims that about 75 percent of all pro basketball players use it.

These drugs will definitely give you a lift. But the aftereffects of their use are severe fatigue and lethargy. Possible side effects are forms of psychosis.

Why do we use them? They offer stimulation, to get a lift, a rise, to overcome fatigue, the blahs, and burn-out. We want energy. People have more confidence in a chemical than in their own ability to control their energy. In essense, they have admitted that they can't do anything about their problems. They must seek the answers outside of themselves. When the kick from cigarettes and alcohol isn't enough, they turn to something stronger, more potent. Also, most statistics indicate a great number of Americans feel they need a lot of chemical help to make it. More than 75 million Americans consume at least one drug a week, most of them every day. Over $2½ billion a year is spent on over-the-counter medications and another $11 billion a year is spent on prescription drugs in the United States.

It is a simple fact: in our search for stimulation, we have allowed tobacco, alcohol, and other mood-altering drugs to become our master. The tragedy is not so much the actual health dangers, but our willingness to admit that we are nothing without the help of a chemical friend. Life is only exciting when we have something artificial to give us a boost. It is that mindset that carries over into our entire outlook on life and that creates a society interested in more and more of whatever turns you on. Even the things we do for enjoyment have become infected with this self-deprecating philosophy.

The All-American Way

Vicariously, we try to experience the ultimate high of winning the World Series with the bases-loaded, bottom-of-the-ninth home run, or playing at a sold-out Madison Square Garden rock concert. And it all started with that natural desire we have to find more energy. Let me illustrate.

In the 1950s, television began to have an impact on the American way of life. Evening meals were scheduled around "Uncle Miltie" and "Our Miss Brooks." By the 1960s 90 percent of American homes had a TV to show them, among other things, morning films of the night before's Vietnam battles, followed by Captain Kangaroo. A full 98 percent of our households boasted of at least one television by the 1970s and it was estimated that average school children watched 3½ hours each day and saw over 250,000 commercials by the time they graduated from high school. If you go back and examine the content of programming over those 30 years, you will notice that each season tries to outdo the last in terms of action.

I do not intend to moralize, but to illustrate the extent to which television has programmed our thinking. When confronted by angry moralists, television producers respond with the seemingly irrefutable truth that "we show only what sells—what the public wants." The fact is, that in our quest for stimulation, we have developed an insatiable desire for more. There is nothing inherently wrong with a soap opera or situation comedy. There is something drastically wrong, however, when that show becomes a fix, mainlining a quick kick to us to get us through the day. Whenever we have to go outside of ourselves for stimulation, we lay ourselves wide open to negative addiction, which could lead to decreased energy. A lifestyle dominated by television viewing can hardly be described as energetic.

Of course, television isn't the only culprit. The need to be stimulated is one reason why spectator-sport attendance remains high even during depressed economic times. Hold on a minute, you say! A day at the old ball park can be a great energizing experience. Here in the Midwest, a favorite fall pastime is a tailgate picnic in the parking lot of a football stadium followed by an exciting collegiate football game. I'm all for it. Yet there is a side to spectator sports that is becoming increasingly ugly: the thirst for violence. Any car race promoter will tell you the best way to assure a packed grandstand is to have an occasional spectacular crash. People are repelled by the sight of blood at a boxing match, but even after the occurrence of an increased number of deaths in the ring in recent years, tickets are selling better than ever. Last year's baseball season set records in attendance, while providing what appeared to be more bench-clearing brawls than ever before. Deacon Jones, former rampaging defensive end for the Los Angeles Rams said it better than I ever could. "Football is meant to be a violent sport, that's what makes it so popular. People want blood. They want toughness. They want violence . . ."

If you think I'm exaggerating this relationship between spectator sports and the need for stimulation, consider the spinoffs spawned by sport. When motorcycle racing became passé, Evel Kneivel burst onto the scene, jumping anything in sight that promised a slight chance of disaster. Olympic-style diving is certainly exciting, but not nearly as appealing as diving from heights of 150 feet, as is done by daredevils on network sports features. Recently, an entire television series was developed that highlighted such danger-filled stunts as driving a car at 90 miles per hour off of a ramp leading into a lake, or being handcuffed to the tracks of a roller coaster due to arrive just milliseconds before the daring performer escaped. Accusations of preplanned disasters and carelessness about the performers' safety have only increased the size of the audience. The obvious answer to the question, "What's next?" was answered frighteningly a few years ago in yet another form of entertainment. The movie "Rollerball" graphically portrayed a society of thrill-seekers queueing up at box offices to see a new breed of athletes physically annihilate one another.

Other forms of entertainment have fallen into this pattern of one-upmanship. Depending on which way you look at it, music has come a long way since the days of baroque chamber recitals and concert hall decorum. Perhaps Elvis got it started with his perpetually undulating lower torso, but he was soon outdone by much sought-after rock acts that feature performers who demonstrate behavior with emphasis upon sadism, masochism, and general vulgarity. In film, slow-motion, stop-action conventional killing has become old hat. Now, slow-motion, stop action *un*conventional killing is in vogue.

I'm sure by now you're beginning to realize just how old-fashioned I really am. Yet the point of all of this is not to offer my bleak judgment on the human race. Regardless of the moral label that you place on modern culture, when you become hopelessly addicted to the role of a spectator, two things happen. First, you have denied yourself the opportunity to be your own stimulating, energizing agent. You have, in effect, declared, "I can no longer find energy in things that I do, only in things that I sit back and watch." Second, you can become vulnerable to a desensitization that allows you to vocally oppose violence and degradation, while still being the first in line when the next freak show arrives in town. You become increasingly vulnerable to the syndrome that causes you to keep chasing thrills until there's nothing left to outdo the last one. The result is a pervasive form of bordom that typifies nonenergetic people. Nothing turns them on any more, hence there is a loss of drive and the resolve to do anything but exist with the faint hope that something thrilling will happen someday.

The Materialism Trap

Living in an affluent society has also given us an illusion of being able to escape that boredom brought on by a dependency on outside elements. Again, the solution to such boredom is found externally. When television fails to provide the stimulus you need, turn it off and turn on your snowmobile, or powerboat, or 4-wheel-drive stump-jumper. It's as much as to say "Give me enough things and I'll be happy."

The materialism trap is one of the most insidious and subtle forms of domination known. It is based on the premise that nothing satisfies. Yet it begins with that dangerous assumption, "If I only had one of those small, nylon backpacking tents and some hiking boots, I'd really be happy." After a few camping trips with this equipment, you opt for the mountaineering model complete with floor and zippered bug screen. The next year, it's a camper, and of course, to pull it you need a bigger car. A few years after that and you may buy a self-contained, air-conditioned, fully carpeted, motor home complete with wet bar and dishwasher. And secretly you're dreaming of owning a private mountain resort.

Indeed, the entire American way of life is programmed toward the accumulation of things, not for the sake of utility, but for the pleasure we get from owning. Few people buy a car with the intention of driving it until it quits running. We buy every two or three years because new cars look better, sound better, and smell better. Similarly, we seldom wear clothes until they wear out. Indeed, patching and darning are almost obsolete activities. We buy clothes to keep up with the styles.

Such a materialistic way of life has awesome moral implications. How can we justify the way we live when over a billion of the world's population is actually starving? Yet the real irony is the end result. Those who live in a simpler, less materialistic culture often are happier, better adjusted, and more energetic people. Those who spend the least amount of time chasing after happiness seem to find it and enjoy it more.

Of course, wealth shouldn't be a whipping post that lets some off the hook while laying the blame at the feet of the rich. Sociologist Dr. Anthony Compolo in his book, *The Success Fantasy*, includes the quest for prestige and power in this syndrome. Many times, wealth has nothing to do with what appears to be a materialistic lifestyle. Instead, individuals try to get their lift from the prestige and power that accompanies traditional success. The typical, aggressive, hostile person will fight to win, whether the prize is money or match sticks. The real goal is the prestige of being an achiever, and a conqueror.

As Bertrand Russell has observed, a life too full of excitement is an exhausting life, "in which continually stronger stimuli are needed to give the thrill that has come to be thought an essential part of pleasure." More recently, psychologist Sam Keen declared that overstimulation of any kind—even a surfeit of entertainment or sexual ecstasy—"destroys the rhythm of health" and "can make us insensitive to the risks and pleasures of ordinary living." When the palate becomes dulled to every kind of pleasure, we end by substituting "titillations for profound organic satisfactions, cleverness for wisdom, and jagged surprises for beauty."

Ours is a culture that leaps at any opportunity to be stimulated. We grope from one fix to the next, hoping to find that elusive, ultimate trip. Our habits of smoking and drinking don't provide it. Our forms of entertainment promise it but never deliver. The things we play with offer little relief from the lethargic boredom that grips us. Yet we keep trying, keep reaching, distraught, dissatisfied, unhappy, and out of gas. What's left?

I know this chapter has been depressing. It wasn't easy to write. I'm a very optimistic person, but I think you need to see why Americans are tired, and what we are doing to ourselves in our attempts to be more energetic. We're chasing false goals. Our best source of energy is ourselves. We have the physical and emotional capabilities to live lives with a maximum of energy, if we are willing to capitalize on our own abilities and make use of current information on building energy.

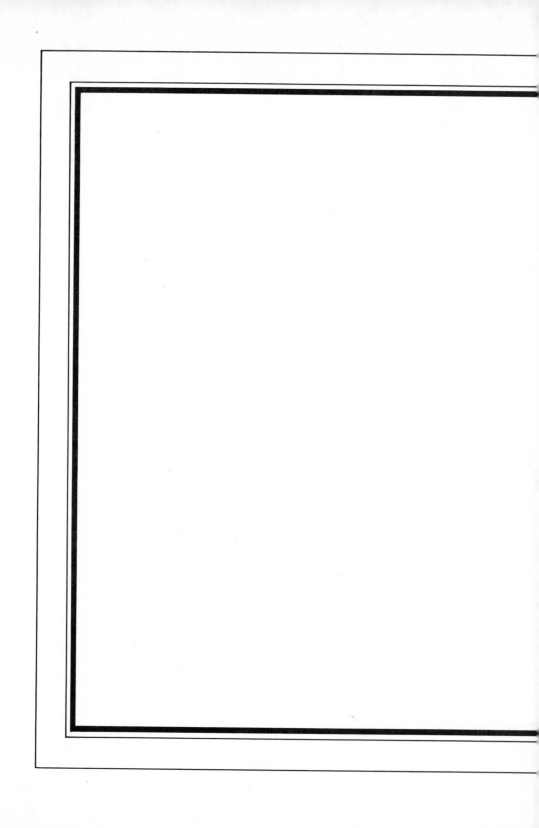

SECTION II: YOUR ENERGY QUOTIENT

CHAPTER 5
Sheer Energy

A panty hose ad sings "sheer energy." A breakfast cereal touts "go power." A beverage company tells you that their soda will leave you "feelin' good." Everyone tells you that their product will give you energy, gusto, and zest for life. You're told you must get your energy from some outside source. But you have read the first four chapters of this book and you no longer believe them. All your energy illusions have been shattered. Now you're hoping I'll give you the facts, the real stuff of energy, the answers.

And I will, but there's one other thing I need to explain first—your American way of living isn't the only factor that you need to consider in assessing your energy level. The other factor is the body you were born with and the internal energy that came with it.

Where does your internal energy come from? Why do some people have more energy than others? Why do you seem to have more energy at one time than at another? And why do some tasks make you sleepy and others energetic? Those $64,000-questions are not easy to answer. One reason is that it's impossible for a scientist to measure your energy level. Yet, every one of us, the scientist included, knows when he does or doesn't have high energy levels. You know both when you're full of energy and when you're not.

To understand energy you must see the phenomenon of your physiology and body chemistry. You must understand what you have to work with to maximize your personal energy.

The Brain

Some experts believe that you get your energy potential from your brain's chemicals and structure. This balance is largely dictated by your genes. Your brain is truly amazing. It weighs slightly more than three pounds and has about 100 billion nerve cells. These nerve cells are extremely tiny but they have a definite structure and function. Structurally, these nerve cells look like a lopsided spider. The "body" of the spider is the cell body. Extending from the cell body are spiderlike arms. The short arms are called dendrites. The single long arm is an axon. The axon's length can be anywhere from a fraction of a millimeter to well over one yard long. These nerve cells with long and short arms are so densely packed and intertwined in your brain that it looks like an electrician's nightmare.

The axons, however, interface with the dendrites of another nerve cell. They are not fastened together, but are separated by a microscopic gap called a synapse. These many nerve cells with dendrites and axons serve as a communications network for the brain and your nervous system. They help transmit impulses throughout the brain quickly and efficiently via a relay mechanism.

A Special Relay Team

When a relay team runs a race, each runner passes a baton to the next runner. The baton is passed in what trackmen call a passing zone. The passing of the baton shows that the runners are close enough so that the "fresh" runner can take over for the "tired" runner. Your neurons, dendrites, synapses, and axons act like a relay team, only an impulse is passed rather than a baton.

The movement of the nerve impulses is electrical in nature. During the passage of the nerve impulse, rapid electro-chemical changes take place along the nerve. The impulse travels from the dendrites toward the axon. When the impulse gets to the end of the axon it must pass over the gap or synapse to the next cell's dendrites. The synapse is much like the passing zone in the relay race. Help is needed to make the jump between the axon of one nerve and the dendrite of another, so a chemical is released that permits the impulse to travel across the synapse. As soon as the impulse is across the synapse, another chemical is released and destroys the activity of the first chemical. This release and destruction of chemicals is very important. It allows for only one message to be transmitted at a time. But the relay pass is successful and the race continues on to the spinal cord, brain, or muscles. All this happens extremely fast.

Nerve Transmitters

The chemicals that transmit the impulse from nerve cell to nerve cell are called nerve transmitters. Many nerve transmitters have been discovered and probably many more will be found in the future.

As you would suspect, these various nerve transmitters are not secreted randomly. Instead, selected nerve cells secrete only one kind of transmitter, such as dopamine, acetylcholine, epinephrine, norepinephrine, or serotonin. By secreting only one kind of chemical the electrical impulse finds its way throughout the maze of cells in the brain. These nerve transmitters make road maps or blueprints for the electrical impulse and the resulting action. Actions include: thinking, talking, walking, singing, loving, writing, moving, hating, and enjoying—in other words, enjoying and celebrating life.

Over the years, scientists have isolated the role of the known chemicals. They know norepinephrine plays a role in dreaming and in your emotions. Dopamine helps you to make coordinated movements.

These nerve transmitters also play a role in your energy levels. Experts tell us that mood swings occur because of too much or not enough chemicals being secreted. For example, if your brain produces too much norepinephrine you may be moved to uncontrollable rage. Likewise, too little production of this chemical may cause the blues or depression.

Of course, mood swings are much more complex than the secretion of one or two chemicals. It is conceivable that selected nerve cells may be oversensitive to certain chemicals. Or the brain may produce the right amount of norepinephrine but the chemical is not removed quickly enough from the synapse. It is also possible that mood shifts may be dependent upon the intensity of the "electrical" surge across the synapse or along the axon.

Regardless of the reason, it can be safely stated that, to a point, your inborn energy levels are dictated by chemicals, electrical impulses, and various nerve cells. Consequently, you may have very high or low energy levels simply because you may or may not secrete a certain amount of nerve transmitters.

The Nervous System

The nervous system itself also plays an important role in your energy levels. Your autonomic nervous system is composed of both the sympathetic and parasympathetic nervous systems. The parasympathetic nervous system is the one that keeps you calm, cool, and collected. It keeps your blood pressure and heart rate low, reduces the secretion of various hormones, and keeps you on an even keel. In other words, it dampens your emotions and reactions to various experiences and events.

The sympathetic nervous system, on the other hand, heightens your response to life's events. It increases your heart rate and blood pressure. It releases more blood sugar into your bloodstream. It secretes extra amounts of hormones so that you can fight for longer periods of time and it speeds up your metabolic rate. Old Fred back in Chapter 3 made it back to the cave in time because of his sympathetic nervous system.

In general, your sympathetic nervous system keeps you wide awake, vital, and full of energy. The activation of the sympathetic nervous system can be good for heightened energy.

It helps you to enjoy the energetic part of your life to the fullest. Without your sympathetic nervous system you would not be able to make love. The winning of a football game could not be savored. There would be little desire or motivation to excel. But if the sympathetic system is activated too often and too long, it can be bad for your energy levels as I will explain later. A fine balance must be kept between the stimulation of the sympathetic and the parasympathetic nervous system for maximum personal energy.

Your brain and nervous system, however, aren't the only sources of energy lifts or letdowns. The endocrine or hormonal system plays a crucial role as well.

The Pituitary Gland

The pituitary gland, the chief activator, is only about ½ inch in diameter and is located at the base of your brain. It has a profound effect on your energy. It activates other glands to action. The pituitary gland secretes many hormones that may influence your growth and the color of your skin. I'll not dwell on these. I'll only concentrate on those pituitary hormones that raise or lower your level of energy.

The pituitary gland secretes ACTH or adrenocorticotropic hormone. ACTH stimulates the adrenal cortex, which activates cortisol, a hormone that has a direct effect on your energy. When you are anticipating a stressful or exciting event, your adrenals will secrete more cortisol. Cortisol levels increase when you're waiting for a test to begin, anticipating your first airplane ride, or getting ready to go down a roller coaster chute. When the event takes place, your cortisol level drops and other hormones take over. Cortisol levels also change throughout the day. When you are concentrating hard to meet a deadline, or you're experiencing an upsetting event such as an argument, or going through an unsure situation, your cortisol levels will rise. Conversely, when everything seems in synchronization, your cortisol level will drop.

The secretion of cortisol is very useful. It prepares you for the impending event by sharpening your senses and gradually introducing you to the excitement of the actual event. By sharpening your senses, you are able to fully appreciate the activity. You have greater feelings of energy. Think of what life would be like without any anticipation or excitement. Our world and life would be dull, dull, dull.

The pituitary gland also secretes thyrotropic—the thyroid-stimulating hormone (TSH). TSH regulates the size and structure of the thyroid and stimulates the production of thyroxine.

Thyroxine

Thyroxine has a profound effect upon your whole body and energy levels. Thyroxine affects what doctors call your metabolism. Your metabolism is the speed with which your body's cells burn the food that you have digested and the oxygen that your body takes in. Each cell is dependent upon oxygen and selected food nutrients to perform its duty, whether that duty is contraction by muscle cells, thinking and reasoning by brain cells, or the transmission of impulses by nerve cells.

If a lot of it is secreted, thyroxine allows the cells of your body to utilize oxygen and nutrients very rapidly. Hence, your metabolism is high. People who have an excessive amount of thyroxine secreted tend to feel jittery, have a rapid heart rate, and increased blood pressure. If your body releases excessively low amounts of thyroxine, the opposite occurs and you are listless and lethargic.

One of the best concrete explanations of a low level of thyroxine and a lack of energy was given by Dr. M. F. Graham. He notes: "Thyroid hormones are essential to the metabolism and combustion of body fuels—sugar and fat. When such fuels are improperly utilized, the result is fatigue, just as an automobile with an improperly adjusted carburetor may run tired."

Normally, thyroxine production is fairly constant and only under stress, pressure, or something similar does your pituitary gland stimulate your thyroid gland to produce more thyroxine. Hence, one of the reasons you feel hyper or jittery during a speech, athletic event, or during an argument is because of your thyroxine level. Much like cortisol, if you didn't produce thyroxine, your life would be boring. Keep remembering that these hormones allow you to enjoy life to its fullest.

Some people, however, have a permanently malfunctioning thyroid gland. Consequently, they are listless or jittery all the time depending upon whether their body produces not enough or too much of the hormone. A person who has a thyroid gland that does not secrete enough thyroxine finds that his metabolism is very slow. Since food is not used at a proper rate, the person becomes fat. An underactive thyroid also produces a feeling of listlessness. It's not that a person is lazy, he just doesn't have the energy to move.

I have a friend, Corrine, who had a tumor on her thyroid gland when she was five. An operation removed the growth, but almost all of her thyroid gland was removed. As a result, she must take thyroid medication each day. Unfortunately, she has struggled with her weight for most of her life. Despite that fact, she is careful about her diet now and runs regularly. Yet her metabolic rate tends to be lower than yours or mine.

An underactive thyroid of this type occurs in only about 2 out of every 100 people who are obese. Consequently, if you have a weight-gain problem, you should not surmise that it's due to a sluggish thyroid. It's probably due to a sedentary lifestyle and improper eating habits.

A person with a sluggish thyroid can be helped with pills made from the thyroids of animals. Doctors, however, should not give this pill unless they've done a careful study and have determined that the patient has a sluggish thyroid.

An overactive thyroid can also cause problems. Here the body burns food too rapidly. Loss of weight and excessive appetite are symptoms of an overactive thyroid. Other signs of the disease are nervousness, lack of sleep, and dizziness. In some instances the eyes bulge and give a person a staring look. Sweating when you should be cold is another symptom. Also, sometimes the thyroid gland becomes enlarged.

There are several factors affecting thyroid production. Some people may be born with a defective gland, or a tumor may appear. It's possible that there may not be enough iodine in the diet. But other reasons are also recognized. Worry, fear, anxiety, and other emotional stresses and strains may be factors. These stress factors can stimulate the production of the thyroid hormone. As a result, the thyroid can be worked to death. The extra stimulation may cause the thyroid to become overactive, and then after a while, it gives up and the person suffers from underactivity.

You may know people who are on some kind of thyroid medication. Sometime, ask them how they feel. Many will tell you that immediately after taking the thyroxine they feel a rush of energy. The rush is followed by a hyped-up feeling. They're jittery. Their pulse rates may be 130 or more beats per minute. As their day wears on, however, the thyroxine level is somewhat modulated and they gradually settle down. Near the end of the day, or 24 hours later, the effectiveness of the medication is waning and they start to get lethargic and experience a downtrodden feeling. That is why most people on thyroxine pills take their medication early in the day. They get the sudden lift early in the morning, much like you get with your coffee. Then, throughout the day they experience more normal levels. They are sleeping when the thyroxine levels are lowest, at night. Corrine takes three thyroid pills a day. At one time she took all in the morning, but she felt much too hyper. So, she switched to early morning, 10:00 A.M., and 2:00 P.M. If she takes the last pill any later, she is too "up" to sleep.

Other Pituitary Hormones

The pituitary secretes two other hormones as well. ADH (an anti-diuretic) and vasopressin. Both of these hormones can raise your blood pressure. Increased blood pressure for an emergency may be good. But if it is increased for an extended period of time, it may adversely affect your energy levels in a rather strange way. Experts theorize that the fatigue which usually accompanies high blood pressure patients may be due to the effort of the body to lower the pressure since blood pressures tend to drop with rest.

The Adrenal Gland

Besides the pituitary gland and its influence on other glands, the adrenal gland plays an important role in your energy levels. This gland secretes a hormone called epinephrine, sometimes called adrenalin. We all know about athletes who say they've got their juices flowing or that their adrenalin is really pumping. Adrenalin increases your blood sugar and speeds up your heart. It can increase your metabolic rate as much as 150 percent or more. People who are given a shot of synthetic adrenalin feel a tremendous rush of energy. They feel capable of doing things they normally couldn't do and become extremely hyper and jittery.

Your own adrenalin can cause you to respond in the same way. When the adrenal glands are stimulated by fear, anger, anxiety, or excitement, an "adrenalin high" is produced. You actually feel a surge. The amount of adrenalin secreted by your adrenal glands is dictated by heredity and the severity of the real or imagined threat.

Adrenalin, therefore, has a dynamic effect on your energy levels. When released, you feel wide awake, alert, and raring to go. Usually fear, stress, and excitement cause this hormone to be secreted. Many athletes seem to be able to will an increase in adrenalin. By concentrating on the event and their competition, they psych themselves "up" for the event. In other words, they're able to deliberately increase their adrenalin levels.

Your Biological Clock

I would like to mention another source of energy that is often overlooked: your biological clock. Each individual seems to have a timing device within them that increases or decreases their supply of energy. That may sound rather complicated, but people's inner clocks differ no more than those of larks, which are active in the day, compared to owls, which are active at night. Allow me to illustrate.

My wife, Beth, is a late evening person. I'm an early morning person. The most creative part of the day for me is before noon. I like to be up by five or six o'clock in the morning because I know my energy levels will be really cranked up. I leave my perfunctory tasks for the afternoon because my motivation and drive is way down. Beth, on the other hand, is just starting to rev her engines by the time I'm winding down. She is extremely energetic in the evening and seems to enjoy more energy as midnight approaches. The next morning, however, she has to start slowly because her level of energy is down.

Everyone has this clock within them, and no one's sure why. The limited research in the area suggests that part of it is inborn and part of it is learned. As far as I'm concerned, that's not the important part. It's far more important that you know when your body produces its greatest amount of energy and try to arrange your activities around the highs and lows. If you are an owl, save your creative work for the evening. If you are a lark, don't try to accomplish major tasks in the late afternoon. By getting your work and activity load in "sync" with your biological clock, you will more fully utilize your energy potential.

The interplay of your nervous system, brain, and hormonal systems illustrates quite clearly how your body can be energized internally. It demonstrates how you can activate resources within your body to increase or decrease your energy levels.

As you would gather, these systems are a double-edged sword. While they can keep you alert, vital, and energized, they can also do you in with respect to fatigue. They can cause you to bottom out. Usually they give you problems when your emotions run rampant, and cause you to decrease your innate energy.

You might be thinking, this is all very interesting, but what can I do about it? The answer is, not much. You could go to your doctor and have some tests taken to determine how much of which hormones you secrete when. But there is little sense in that. I don't recommend taking any drugs to supplement your hormone production unless you have exhausted the suggestions given in the rest of this book. Relying on medication slips you back into dependency on some exterior source. It also could quickly become a serious negative addiction that would throw your system completely out of whack. It is conceivable that your hormones are the source of your energy problem, but I doubt it. Instead, consider the other possible options. The next chapter will help you to learn where and how to begin.

CHAPTER 6
Your Life Space

Two Stories

The year was 1928. Hulda Crooks was tired; and I mean tired. She had just finished a grueling number of years in which she had moved from her rural farm in Canada, belatedly finished her high school education, attended Loma Linda University in California, and received her degree in dietetics. Adding to this intense activity was the fact that she worked her way through both high school and college.

She also married Dr. Samuel A. Crooks, instructor of anatomy at Loma Linda University. She was in love. But she was also pooped. "He literally took me for better or worse," she confided. Working for her college degree had worn her out. She remembers, "I wasn't worth much. I was nervous, anemic, and perpetually tired. As I worked for my support and education, year after year of indoor life took its toll. So, although I gained an education I lost my health and energy. I was so tired, I was afraid I would die."

She was only in her late 20s but she was exhausted. She was too tired to cook, work, or think. Life scared her. The grim reaper seemed around the corner.

Hulda's new husband started her on a plan to help her get back her energy and vitality. She was to spend as much time outdoors as possible, gardening and raising lovebirds, calves, and goats. She was also to improve her mind, develop a positive attitude about life, and follow a healthful, vegetarian eating plan.

Another perfect antidote was her husband's encouragement to return to the outdoors that she had learned to love as a child. Outdoors she had energy.

Outdoors she had strength. She even gave her home the appearance of out-doors. At first she could barely walk around the block. But as time progressed she was able to walk for miles, and work for hours in the yard.

As Hulda's strength and vitality started to return she began to do more demanding things. Backpacking and mountain climbing became a way of life. Expeditions would last from one to six weeks. Vacations were spent at altitudes of 11,000 feet.

By the time I met and interviewed Hulda she was 84 years old and far from ready for the rocking chair. She was sweet, alert, vibrant, and energetic, a real "possibility" thinker. As we chatted, she told me that she still was an avid backpacker. She had climbed Mt. Whitney 18 times in the past 18 years. In 1972 she crossed the Sierra Nevada range from Sequoia to Whitney Portal—an 80-mile trip. In 1974 she completed the 212-mile John Muir Trail, over a period of five summers. And at the age of 81 she started working on the Sierra Club's list of 268 peaks. Now she has over 50 peaks to her credit, in altitudes up to 11,500 feet.

She began to run at the age of 70. Today she has run distances of up to a half marathon (13.1 miles). Starting in 1977 she gave the Senior Olympics a shot. During that year she placed first in the 1,500-meter run. She returned in 1978 to totally dominate the senior track world. First she won the 800 meters, with a time of 5:48 (5 minutes, 48 seconds). Then she won the 1,500 meters in 10:59. Finally, she won the 5,000 meters in 39:49, a new record for her age group.

Sitting and listening to her was a treat. I felt I was in the presence of one of the world's special people. I left her small apartment feeling good about life, getting older, and people. I was energized.

Steve McKanic had also virtually run out of steam. After 22 years of building a nice fuel oil delivery business, his lifestyle had caught up with him. Skipping breakfast, gulping coffee, smoking 3½ packs of cigarettes a day, and working 18-hour-days had just about done him in. Each day he found it more and more difficult to drag himself out of bed and off to work. Finally, the "big one" hit and laid him flat in a hospital. The prognosis was bleak. Couched in medical jargon, the doctor told Steve they could do nothing. His heart was too diseased for bypass surgery. Two cardiologists at separate medical schools told him, "No hope. Go home, get your things in order. At most you have six months to live. In fact, if you want to live that long, take this medication and stay in bed."

Steve's back was to the wall and he knew it. At first, Steve moped around the house cursing his fate. He spent a lot of time "if onlying." You know, "If only I had taken it easier. If only I had gone on a diet." When he tired of that, he made a decision. He vowed that if he was going to die it would be in the saddle, not in a rocking chair.

He began reading vigorously about heart disease, to learn what he could do. His conclusion was: fight back.

- Develop a positive attitude about life.
- Lose 80 pounds.
- Stop smoking 3½ packs of cigarettes a day.
- Begin exercising.
- Improve eating habits. That is, less fat, sugar, and salt. And supplement the diet with vitamins and minerals.

Gradually, Steve became a new person. One night he even went for a walk. He did it late at night so no one could see him. His wife was upset. At the end of the walk he was mildly surprised that nothing happened. So he went for another walk the next day, fully expecting to drop dead. He didn't, so he continued the next, and the next, and the next.

Steve couldn't believe it. The more he walked the better he felt. He joined a fitness class and even started running. Over the months, he moved up to walking and jogging 10 to 11 miles a day. This gave him more energy than he'd ever thought possible.

His weight started to drop. His nutrition improved dramatically. He did two other things that shocked many—he flushed his medicine down the toilet and refused to see doctors anymore. He thought their approach was too negative.

Steve didn't stop with these efforts. He spent eight hours a day for a year studying how to improve his health. He took courses at a local college in nutrition, fitness, psychology, and stress management. He added one more element as well. He started to share his newfound information with friends and strangers. When someone had a heart attack he visited them in the hospital and told them there was hope, or could be, if they began assuming responsibility for their own health. He encouraged them to get the most out of what they had left AND never give up.

Steve lived for more than seven years after his April 1973 heart attack. He told me just before his death in July 1980 that the last seven years of his life were his best. He gave and received more energy, fun, and love during those years than all of his previous 47 years combined. Steve was special, and he illustrates an important point: even if you already have one foot in the grave, it's not too late to achieve your maximum remaining energy potential.

These stories are important. You simply must not count yourself too old or too far gone to do something about your lack of healthful energy. Hulda and Steve had every reason to give up. I've seen many who have given up. They figure there is no use, so they continue doing things that destroy their energy levels. They sit and mope and complain about their lot in life. And their energy levels falter. It's sad, because it doesn't have to be that way, for them or for you. So let's begin with today—now.

The first thing you must do is recognize that you're responsible for your own behavior, feelings, actions, and attitudes. You must learn to take charge of yourself. You're the person responsible for how you act and feel. You can change your actions—if you decide to do so.

The hardest thing you will need to learn is how to overcome immobilization. Immobilization may range from mild indecision to total inaction. Here are some examples:

- You don't exercise because you're afraid you won't have the time.
- You want to exercise but are afraid people will laugh at you.
- You want to eat salad at noon but are afraid your associates will make fun of your "light" lunch.
- You suffer from high blood pressure because you are dissatisfied with your lot in life—family, job, and social.
- You want to stop taking Valium because you think it makes you "spacy" but your doctor feels that it's helping you.
- You would like to meditate or offer a prayer at a restaurant, but are afraid people will stare at you when your head is bowed.
- You avoid talking to someone, yet you realize that a few words would open up a new relationship.
- You have a difficult time introducing yourself to someone who intrigues and fascinates you.
- You don't want to drink alcoholic beverages but find it extremely difficult and embarrassing to say "No thank-you, I don't drink."

Immobilization, as far as I'm concerned, is a great energy-waster. You can spend an inordinate amount of time worrying and deciding what is best to do.

That means you accomplish very little. You will live a more energetic life if you break away from this pattern of inaction and begin to attack the things that bother you.

Think back to when you were a youngster. Perhaps you weren't doing all the studying that you should have been doing for your school work. You knew you were going to get a poor grade. The anxiety of waiting for your report card was almost too much to bear. You felt lousy. You wanted to sleep most of the time and avoid confrontation with your family.

Physically, your body was reacting. Your hormones and nervous systems were being overstimulated and, soon, fatigue set in. Maybe you couldn't feel better until you talked the problem out. Action reduced your anxiety. Action today can do the same kind of thing. It gives you a sense of direction and purpose and reduces your anxiety.

Of course, no one can move you to action. To paraphrase the old adage, I can lead you to water but you must decide to drink it for yourself. Increased personal energy is indeed an individual responsibility. Once you understand that personal energy is your job and that action is important, it's time for you to take stock of your current life space. Where are you right now? It is imperative that you examine yourself before starting any program of improvement. That's one of my many complaints regarding all the popular diets. They rush you headlong into a crash program of all this and none of that, without assessing your nutritional needs. You may find that poor nutrition is the key to your energy problem. Or your problem may be stress. Possibly it's obesity. Quite probably, it's a combination. The point is, you need to know what concerns you the most. Then you need to begin there. Zero in on the one area that concerns you most. Then begin your trek to more energy by working on that problem.

Avoid the pitfall of trying to change all your behaviors at once. People who try to give up smoking and coffee at the same time, and then start exercising as well, usually are not successful. It's best if you do one thing and do it well. When you have experienced success in one area and feel good about what you have done, then move on to another area of concern. There's nothing like some success to bring on more success. Also, tackle an area that is most pressing to you, one you really want to change. Don't try to change one that someone else is nagging you about. Your chances for success will be far greater this way than if you pick some area that you feel lukewarm about.

I have a good friend who every New Year's Eve made a resolution to give up smoking, cut back on his coffee, start exercising, and lose 15 pounds. He was filled with excellent intentions, but the change was too dramatic. He tried for about two weeks and then he could no longer stand it. He slipped back into one of his old habits. He started to feel bad that he blew it. His self-esteem dropped and soon he had thrown the baby out with the wash water and picked up his negative addictions all over again.

This past year I convinced him to pick out one area and get that under control. I suggested that his change should be something positive. I told him not to focus on his negative addictions of smoking and drugs. Instead I wanted him to focus on positive things such as exercise and meditation. It's my position that negative addictions will disappear when positive addictions become commonplace in your life.

My friend chose exercise. He decided to spend 30 minutes a day walking. Progress was slow at first. But by mid-July he was jogging and putting in two to three miles every other day. At the end of the summer, when I was putting the finishing touches on this book, he came to me and said, "You know, Charlie, I've dropped about seven pounds even though I didn't pay attention to my diet and have continued to exercise. Now, I think I'm ready to cut back on my coffee."

I think my friend's approach is best. Trying to do everything at once is counterproductive. It's like trying to learn several new languages at one time.

A Lifelong Process

Another important point is that you must understand that building energy is a lifelong process. Make changes when you are good and ready for them. It's an evolving process, and dynamic as well. You make commitments, evaluate those changes, and then decide to keep, change, or modify as you experience new energy-building techniques.

Here's a brief summary of my own commitment to building energy.

Age	Energy Building Stages
13	Exercised regularly, including 1 to 3 miles of running per day.
14–17	Developed strong self-concept to do things physically.
22	Cut back on salting my food.
22–28	Developed strong self-concept or ability to do things intellectually.
27	Reduced sugar consumption.
	Spiritual awakening.
29	Reduced saturated fat content in my diet.
31	Increased my distance running to 4 to 5 miles a day.
32	Developed and practiced neuromuscular relaxation techniques.

33	Decided not to use medication of any type.
34	Long-distance mileage increased to 6 miles and up.
35	Supplemented my diet with vitamins.
	Discovered that I liked myself.
37	Dropped neuromuscular relaxation techniques and picked up relaxation response and body-scanning techniques.
	Cut back on red meat consumption.
38	Decided to use medication for allergies.
39	Started mineral supplementation.
	Dedicated myself to helping others.
	Flirted with vegetarianism.
40	Returned to meat eating 1 to 2 days each week.

A close look shows you that I made changes when I was ready. Also, I made selected changes when I had to reevaluate my previous decision. For example, I swore off all kinds of medication and yet my allergies plagued me so I resorted to the use of some over-the-counter medication to help me through extremely difficult times. I found that the vegetarian diet I selected was not really satisfactory and pleasurable to me. So I went back to eating red meats once or twice a week.

The point is that the decision to make changes is a dynamic and lifelong process, one that can go in any direction. Building personal energy is not something you do overnight. It's a maturation process. You come to an understanding of your body, mind, and spirit. And that takes time. Don't try to do everything at once. It won't work.

The simple checklist that you'll find in Table 6-1 may help you define the area you should work on. It gives you an idea where you are. It can tell you what you should work on and where you'll probably have the greatest success and then be able to move on. I wish I'd had one of these when I started my whole idea of energy living. It would have kept me from going down too many blind alleys.

The place to start is with the simple self-assessment. The checklist has six areas: Enjoying Life, Enjoying Exercise, Eating Well, Staying Slim, Relating to Others, and Taking Care of Yourself. These areas make up the various category in Section III: Mastery of Skills for maximum personal energy. This checklist will give you an idea of what areas you are doing well in and the areas in which you feel you need help. It will help crystalize your maximum personal energy goals and program.

Once you have identified your major area of concern you are then to follow the principles outlined in the respective section of Section III. For example, if you decide to work on Enjoying Life, Fighting Back, (Chapter 7), The Three Rs, (Chapter 8), and A Three Phase Plan for Enjoying Life should be followed. When you have reached a satisfactory level on the Three Phase Plan, you can then progress to another area of concern.

I tried to avoid generalizations on this self-assessment. If I asked you how you felt about your energy level, you would say, "Oh, pretty good," or "Not so hot." That may make for good conversation but it doesn't give you a handle —something to hold on to. To really get to the root of your energy problem, go over these questions carefully. Perhaps they will stimulate other ideas that you can add to the sheet.

You'll notice that this test has no right or wrong answers. The purpose is to show you what you need to work on to improve your energy. You may find that your level of aerobic fitness is high and that you are satisfied with it. So don't worry about aerobic fitness. On the other hand, you may find that your nutrition is horrible, yet it doesn't bother you. You're satisfied with being a junk-food junkie. You're not convinced it's even a problem. No sense in trying to work on that. Somewhere, however, I'm sure you'll find an area that troubles you. Perhaps it's trying to stay slim. You may even have a relatively high achievement level there, but still you're not satisfied. That's where you want to start because your motivation will be the strongest there.

Your Self-Assessment

To get started, look over Table 6-1. After a brief introduction, you'll find six statements. Read each one carefully, then circle a number on the left that best describes your level of achievement. Be truthful, yet fair. Then, check the box on the right that indicates your level of satisfaction. Are you pleased with your level of achievement, or do you think you need to improve? Again, be honest. If you scored poorly in a given area, yet you really are satisfied to stay at that level, admit it. Remember, this is for you only. No one has to know what you think of yourself—except you.

Checklist Review

Now go over your responses on the right and pinpoint those areas where you feel you need improvement. That's where you need to start in your quest for more energy. Maybe you even want to turn ahead to a chapter that deals with an area that you feel is most urgent. That's fine. You're the boss. (How-

Text Continues on Page 61

TABLE 6-I
Maximum Personal Energy Self Test

Enjoying Life

Enjoyment and energy are like strawberries and cream. They complement each other. If your daily routine has degenerated into mere existence, perhaps you need to evaluate your own attitudes and expectations. Sometimes we get out of life just what we expect. How about you?*

Level of Achievement		Level of Satisfaction		
Low High		OK	Needs Improvement	Could Be Improved But Not a Concern at This Time
1 2 3 4 5	1. I like to find time to be quiet and relax.	☐	☐	☐
1 2 3 4 5	2. I like to express myself in art, music, dance, sports, and hobbies.	☐	☐	☐
1 2 3 4 5	3. I can accept all of my feelings such as being mad, sad, glad, and frightened.	☐	☐	☐
1 2 3 4 5	4. I am often happy, and I find it easy to laugh.	☐	☐	☐
1 2 3 4 5	5. When I make mistakes I admit them and learn from them.	☐	☐	☐
1 2 3 4 5	6. I can tell when I am reacting to stress and have a plan for reducing that stress.	☐	☐	☐

Enjoying Exercise

Becoming physically fit is a tremendous boost to energy. The person who is fit can work eight hours at the office and still have plenty of "go" left over to enjoy an active life at home, in the garden, on the golf course, or with a hobby. Just how do you rate?

*Source: Based on some of the work done by Robert Allen, Ph.D., and the Frost Valley YMCA staff.

Table 6-1—Continued

Level of Achievement		Level of Satisfaction		
		OK	Needs Improvement	Could Be Improved But Not a Concern at This Time
Low High				
1 2 3 4 5	1. I bike, swim, run, or walk for at least 30 minutes, 3 or more times a week.	☐	☐	☐
1 2 3 4 5	2. Whenever possible, I walk or ride a bike instead of using cars, elevators, escalators, etc.	☐	☐	☐
1 2 3 4 5	3. I do some form of stretching several times per week.	☐	☐	☐
1 2 3 4 5	4. I participate in sports for reasons other than competition.	☐	☐	☐
1 2 3 4 5	5. It is fun for me to be physically active.	☐	☐	☐
1 2 3 4 5	6. I try to learn one new sport every two years.	☐	☐	☐

Eating Well

An engine needs a steady supply of good, clean fuel in order to run efficiently. So do you. Food provides that fuel, and like the engine, your body needs a regular supply of good, nutritious food. Too much of this or too little of that will drain your energy supply. Is that something you need to work on?

Level of Achievement		Level of Satisfaction		
		OK	Needs Improvement	Could Be Improved But Not a Concern at This Time
Low High				
1 2 3 4 5	1. I eat a balanced diet and enjoy a variety of fresh, natural foods.	☐	☐	☐
1 2 3 4 5	2. I try to eat foods with little added sugar, salt, and/or saturated fat.	☐	☐	☐
1 2 3 4 5	3. I take time to relax and enjoy my meals. I also eat my food in one location (at a table).	☐	☐	☐

Table 6-1—Continued

Level of Achievement						Level of Satisfaction		
								Could Be Improved But
							Needs	Not a Concern
Low			High			OK	Improvement	at This Time
1 2 3 4 5					4. I consume very little coffee, colas, or other foods high in caffeine.	☐	☐	☐
1 2 3 4 5					5. I eat three well-balanced meals a day—breakfast, lunch, and dinner.	☐	☐	☐
1 2 3 4 5					6. My diet contains a relatively low amount of fat (30 percent or less), a moderate to low amount of meat, and regular portions of complex carbohydrates.	☐	☐	☐

Staying Slim

Staying slim involves a balance between your physical activity and eating behaviors. To have a low percentage of fat and your weight under control, you must select big muscle activities such as walking, running, bicycling, and swimming. You should also build extra activities into your day. That is, never lie down when you can sit, never sit when you can stand, never stand when you can walk. These physical activities should also be complemented with good eating practices.

Level of Achievement						Level of Satisfaction		
								Could Be Improved But
							Needs	Not a Concern
Low			High			OK	Improvement	at This Time
1 2 3 4 5					1. I bike, swim, run, or walk for at least 30 minutes, three or more times a week.	☐	☐	☐
1 2 3 4 5					2. Whenever possible, I walk or ride a bike instead of using cars, elevators, escalators, etc.	☐	☐	☐
1 2 3 4 5					3. I eat foods high in nutrients and low in calories.	☐	☐	☐

Table 6-1—Continued

Level of Achievement						Level of Satisfaction		
Low				High		OK	Needs Improvement	Could Be Improved But Not a Concern at This Time
1	2	3	4	5	4. I eat three meals a day—breakfast, lunch, and dinner.	☐	☐	☐
1	2	3	4	5	5. I don't eat when I'm bored or under pressure.	☐	☐	☐
1	2	3	4	5	6. I cannot pinch more than an inch of fat on my body.	☐	☐	☐

Relating to Others

A few years ago, it wasn't unusual to hear someone say, "Boy, she really gets me down!" That was a good description of how poor relationships can physically sap your strength. Nobody likes to fight or argue. The effects on energy are total: emotional and physical energy is lost. How well do you relate?

Level of Achievement						Level of Satisfaction		
Low				High		OK	Needs Improvement	Could Be Improved But Not a Concern at This Time
1	2	3	4	5	1. I enjoy my family and get along well with my family members.	☐	☐	☐
1	2	3	4	5	2. I can make and maintain friendships.	☐	☐	☐
1	2	3	4	5	3. I try to listen to others without always thinking of what I want to say.	☐	☐	☐
1	2	3	4	5	4. I would rather talk to someone about how I feel than keep it inside.	☐	☐	☐
1	2	3	4	5	5. I am open to people who are different than I (age, race, religion, and interests).	☐	☐	☐
1	2	3	4	5	6. I am able to give and receive love.	☐	☐	☐

Table 6-1—Continued
Taking Care of Yourself

There are many kinds of things we can do in an effort to get energy. We smoke, do drugs, abuse alcohol, take unnecessary risks, and watch violence and mayhem for stimulation. These activities put the emphasis on something outside of you for a lift. These are negative addictions, as Dr. William Glasser, author of *Positive Addiction*, calls them. Ultimately they can drag you down.

Below is a checklist to see how you're doing on these behaviors. But there is one radical difference. Here, however, you will not find a section in Part III on Taking Care Of Yourself. I do not tell you how to stop these behaviors. That's because I know that if you opt for the other positive addictions listed in the book—that is learning how to enjoy life, participating in aerobic exercise, eating good food, staying slim, and relating well to others—there will be no need for your negative addictions. I want you to emphasize the positive.

Level of Achievement		Level of Satisfaction		
Low High		OK	Needs Improvement	Could Be Improved But Not a Concern at This Time
1 2 3 4 5	1. I do not smoke cigarettes.	☐	☐	☐
1 2 3 4 5	2. I *rarely* (not more than once every 2 months) take self-prescribed medicine, i.e., aspirin-type products, suppositories, and other over-the-counter drugs.	☐	☐	☐
1 2 3 4 5	3. I drink 1 to 2 ounces of alcohol or less daily.	☐	☐	☐
1 2 3 4 5	4. I make up my own mind about drug and alcohol use, despite what others are doing.	☐	☐	☐
1 2 3 4 5	5. I ask my physician on the necessity of my taking medication prescribed for me.	☐	☐	☐
1 2 3 4 5	6. I find I am not dependent on external stimuli (drugs, alcohol, cigarettes, sugar, and thrill activities) to get me high.	☐	☐	☐

ever, I would like you to read the entire book.) Regardless, you're the only one that can get the ball rolling. Just do me a favor and attack the problem systematically.

Planning for Energy

To begin, I suggest that you have a plan of action rather than try to do everything at once. The following steps may help you.

Admit Your Problem

This is perhaps one of the most difficult steps to any plan of action. It's also the most necessary. Unless you admit you have a problem, you will never solve it. Table 6-1 is a good place to start. It will show you those areas in which you think you have a problem. The right-hand column labeled "Level of Satisfaction" is the most important part of that survey. You may score yourself rather low in the area of making and maintaining friendships, but as far as you're concerned, that's just fine with you. You see no reason for improvement. That means that as far as you're concerned, you don't have a problem. Your neighbor might perceive it to be a problem. Your husband may perceive it to be a problem. I might perceive it to be a problem. But if it doesn't bother you, there is no sense in trying to change it. You must *admit* that you are too fat, eat poorly, don't get along well with others, or whatever, before you can be successful in correcting any of these areas. Once you have selected an area you can comfortably admit is a problem, you're ready for the next step.

Decide to Change

It's one thing to admit your problem, it's another thing to make the decision to do something about it. How many times have you heard one of your smoking friends declare, "One of these days I've got to quit smoking these things."? That's the way we think when it comes to doing something about our energy problem. The truth is, many of us know that there are areas in which we need some help. Yet we placate ourselves by thinking that all we need to do is go on a crash diet, start to jog, try to get to bed earlier, or take time to learn a hobby or read a book. As you know, it just doesn't happen that way. You need to make a conscious decision that you want to do something about your energy level.

One thing you may have noticed as you considered your life space was the fact that everything else seems to control what you do. You are no longer the one in charge. External factors dominate to such an extent that you perceive your present condition to be one of acquiescence. The only way to break away is to select one area and make a conscious choice to resume control and change that situation. When you begin seeing progress in that area, select another problem and approach it in the same positive way.

Take Stock of Your Condition

The survey gave you a general idea of what sort of problem areas may contribute to your lack of energy. Once you have selected an area that you can admit presents a problem to you, and have decided to do something about that problem, you need to be specific and evaluate your problem. For example, let's say that you are not satisfied with your eating patterns. You have decided to change the way you eat. You select Item #3 under "Eating Well" as an area that needs improvement. You simply do not take time to relax and enjoy your meals and you eat your food on the run or in front of the television. You would like to do something about that.

Taking stock of that problem involves a closer look at mealtime. Why don't you take the time to relax and enjoy meals? What causes you to hurry? How much time is actually spent at the meal table? What sort of activities are taking place while you are eating? Answering these questions will help you to pinpoint the reason why this has become a problem in your particular life space. The key to this step is to take a look at that problem to see if you can figure out how it developed into a problem in the first place. Once you begin to see the causes, you can develop ways to minimize it.

Planning the Attack, Getting Started, and Sticking to It

This is really the fun part, the action part. Just doing something will probably be an energy lift. You are overcoming inertia. I'll not take you through all the steps here because Chapter 18—Getting to Your Goals—does it for you. Just remember that after going through the first three steps you'll have selected an area that you have admitted is a problem. You want to change and have discovered some reasons for that problem existing in your life space. You'll also probably have a huge list of excuses.

I suppose I could fill a book with the excuses people have given for not doing something about their energy level. For example, with exercise it's usually too hot or it's too cold. I'm too fat. I'm too weak. I don't have the time, and so on. Yet as far as I'm concerned, there's only one valid excuse for being slaves to a lack of energy: "I choose not to do anything about it."

When we strip away all of the rationalizations, we uncover the real reason why people do not effectively change. If you really want to do something, you will find a way to do it. In short, you choose to do it. Approach energy in the same way. If you choose to live an energetic life, you will.

I'm sure you've heard all the adages. "There's no time like the present. Don't wait for tomorrow, for tomorrow may never come. Don't put off for tomorrow what you can do today." They may all sound corny, but it's good advice. The sooner you get started incorporating your plan, the sooner you will start seeing the results.

My suggestion now is to read each of the following sections. Don't skim over any unless you now know *exactly* what you want to change in your life. After you've completed reading this book, take the test in Table 6-1 again. It's possible that new information has made you change your opinion on what area you really need to emphasize. After completing this reevaluation, read the pertinent chapter again carefully. Then review the goal-setting chapter and get going. When you achieve a desirable level, move on to a new area of concern.

Once you begin to see some progress, no one will stop you—they won't have the energy.

Now You're Ready

The next section of this book (Section III) gives you a practical plan for retrieving lost energy and discovering new sources of vitality. For each of the five master skills (Enjoying Life, Enjoying Fitness, Eating for Energy, Slimming for Energy, and Relating to Others), you will have two chapters of explanation followed by a Three Phase Plan. By following these plans, you will begin to master the corresponding skills and recover lost energy. The first phase of each plan is a beginner's level. For most people, the beginner's level is the best place to start, even if you think you have mastered that particular area. The second phase of each plan will help you to maintain an energetic lifestyle. For many, the second phase will provide enough energy to satisfy. The third phase will be very difficult to achieve. It will give you the highest amount of energy. It is a good goal to shoot for, but don't get discouraged if it takes you quite a while to get there.

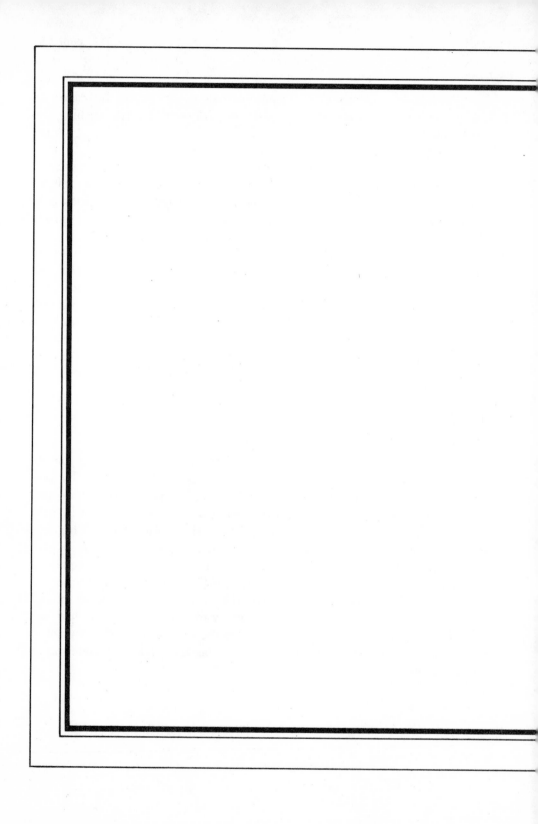

SECTION III: MASTERY OF SKILLS

ENJOYING LIFE

CHAPTER 7
Fighting Back

You've learned that not handling stress properly can ruin your maximum personal energy. Norman was a perfect example. You've also learned that you can fight back—if you want to. Steve McKanic and Hulda Crooks proved that. But to do it you need skills and strategies that work.

For years, psychologists have used the term "coping" to demonstrate an ability to survive and handle today's pressures and changes. I've used it extensively. While the term is good, Dr. Wayne Dyer has convinced me that a better term is "mastery." Coping implies just getting by. Mastery implies that you're in charge. I like that. Therefore, I want to give you some mastery skills that you can use to enjoy life to its fullest.

Scheduling Time

The ability to effectively schedule your time is an important skill in preventing stress from depleting your supply of energy. In fact, you may have read previous suggestions from other authors and complained, "Good things to do, but I just don't have the time or energy to do them." Usually that's due to the fact that many people have not assumed control over the day. Instead, they literally run through a busy list of things to do, try to do them all at once, and hope to someday get "a little room to breathe." Life is busy for everyone. Yet the ones who always seem to have room to breathe are the ones who have learned to manage their time efficiently.

Applying time management techniques in professional and personal life strikes some people as an oppressive prospect calculated to add more stress to an already pressured existence. Time management consultants such as Alan Lakein, however, see the more efficient use of hours and minutes as a way to liberation. From the day you develop and implement a time-use plan, they say, you won't be working harder but working smarter. As a result, the busy person will be able to achieve goals at work and in private life more efficiently and have more time for unstructured activities that can be enjoyed more freely.

Basically, you need to look at your day in terms of four areas: work, sleep, relaxation, and family and social obligations. Obviously, your working segment is pretty much determined for you. That is, work takes up approximately eight hours of each weekday. It is important that before you accept a job, you have a very definite idea of how much time is expected from you.

Write down a schedule for work and try to follow it, making a point of doing the most important or difficult things first. Make small decisions promptly, reminding yourself that in most matters any decision is better than no decision. Be sure to use all the help available to you, delegating work when it is more efficient to do so, and learn to say no when others are in a position to do a piece of work more efficiently and effectively than you.

Alan Lakein suggests listing top goals for both the short term (six months) and long term (lifetime), then listing activities that will take you toward these goals. The idea is to put an A, B, or C next to each according to its importance (if the list is long, A_1, A_2, A_3, etc., may be used). An A activity (or part of one, starting with the easiest or most important task) should be done first each day, preferably early in the day, to be followed by Bs, and if time permits, by Cs. A new list of priorities can be drawn up at the beginning or end of each day to reflect changes in emphasis. A goals for the week ahead can be prepared on Friday afternoon. Lifetime goals, based on the day-to-day and weekly goals, can be mapped at longer intervals. Time each day can be set aside to get in at least one A_1 task for one or more long-range goal.

For overwhelmed people who worry about never getting to their C tasks, Lakein cites what he calls the 80/20 rule: "If all items are arranged in order of value, 80 percent of the value would come from only 20 percent of the items, while the remaining 20 percent of the value would come from 80 percent of the items." Because this rule applies about 80 percent of the time (!), Lakein urges his clients to avoid the tendency to do C tasks, which are usually simpler and therefore more tempting than the vital As. The Cs are relatively insignificant anyway and if they are postponed, it is likely that the need to do some of them at least may disappear as time passes.

There are a number of ways this strategy can be implemented. I use what I call the "three-drawer concept." In my office desk there are three drawers.

My A tasks go in the top drawer, my B tasks go in the middle drawer, and my C tasks go in the bottom drawer. If I had a fourth drawer it would be a waste basket.

This same concept may be applied to personal as well as professional priorities. For example, if you have just had a flat on your car, you have the choice of purchasing a new set of tires as a top drawer priority, or risk being stranded somewhere without a spare. But if your mechanic casually mentioned at your last tune-up that the fan belt is beginning to show some wear, you might consider that a bottom drawer priority. If you get around to replacing it some time before leaving on vacation, that's soon enough.

Another Lakein suggestion is to sort through goals originally classified as Bs and reclassify them as As or Cs. Cs—especially C_2s—can be kept in a file folder in a drawer and reviewed periodically for action or disposal. At first reading, incoming mail can be sorted into folders labeled Action, Information, and Deferred and given appropriate priority on the daily list. As an added help in becoming more efficient, those using the Lakein approach are urged to frequently ask themselves "Lakein's Question"—"What is the best use of my time right now?"

The next area, sleep, may need some special attention. Often, sleep gets pushed out of our schedules. We go to great lengths to avoid being late to work, but if we are late to bed, we don't worry about it. Since a proper amount of sleep is pivotal to abundant energy, you may need to adjust your daily schedule so that you get to bed on time. For most people, six hours of sleep is an absolute minimum. Your own demands may be higher. If so, don't ignore those demands. While it may seem that going to bed an hour earlier cuts into your list of things to do, you will get more done in a shorter period of time if your body is sufficiently rested.

So if you spend eight hours at work, and seven hours sleeping, that leaves nine hours for fun and games, right? Of course not. You've got to mow the lawn, repair the leaky faucet, go shopping, take the kids to the dentist, pay the bills, and everything else. And that's where proper scheduling comes in, because you really *do* have to do all of these things, and more. But you do not have to do all of these things at once. Follow Lakein's advice again or try this: make a list of all those social and household obligations that aren't connected with your job, but must be done. Beside each one, put an approximate amount of time it takes to do them. Now underline those that are absolutely necessary and put a question mark after the ones that could be omitted. Using this list as a guide, make a schedule for each day of the week, setting aside a time for each of the "absolute activities." If there are not enough hours in the week to get everything done, cross out the ones that are followed with question marks. Make sure you include time for relaxation and enjoyment. Then, tape the schedule in a place where you'll see it often, and follow it rigidly for one week. I think you'll find that it works. Why? Because often we put things off until the last minute. Then when it's time to do them, we're in a rush. The task seems extremely unpleasant. That means more stress. We get frustrated. Mope around. Waste time. That's more stress; less energy. On the other hand, by trying to schedule your time on a more orderly basis, you learn that being in control gives a tremendous sense of satisfaction and accomplishment. Those are great allies in your battle for more energy.

Positive Mental Outlook

David Fink, M.D., a psychiatrist who has done extensive work in the area of stress and nervous tension, refers to the "play spirit" of man or woman. In counseling his patients who are troubled, he encourages them to take the play spirit into everything they do. That is, approach each activity as if it were going to be playful and fun. While that may sound simplistic, the concept is important. The attitude with which we approach a situation often dictates how that situation affects us. If you go to work with a feeling of dread or boredom, the chances are you'll get just that.

So my first recommendation is to change your outlook. When you get up in the morning, tell yourself, "Today is going to be a great day!" Approach each task that faces you in a new light. Look for things that are amusing. Try to avoid negative thoughts by replacing them with positive ones. Here are some examples.

Negative	Positive
1. I just don't want to go to work today.	1. Wow, with unemployment so high, I'm sure glad I've got a job.
2. Well, another fruitless trip to the unemployment office.	2. Sure wish I had a job, but I'm glad I live in a country that helps the unemployed.
3. If he says one more thing about my cooking I'm going to scream.	3. Crazy George! Sure he complains a lot, but he's so sweet to me when he gets a chance to relax.
4. This traffic is unbearable. Why do I have to work in this lousy city?	4. I wonder how many drivers I can get to smile and wave at me while I wait in this traffic jam?

5. Not another sleepless night. I
   can't take it!

5. Finally, I have a chance to do
   some reading in peace and quiet.

Okay, enough of the pep talks. I know it doesn't always work this way. But you'd be surprised how a more positive approach to a wearisome situation can turn the experience into a pleasant one.

Getting into the play spirit will help, but obviously it's only the beginning. After all, you need a little play occasionally to keep that positive attitude. According to Fink, play is anything you do that you can drop as soon as it ceases to amuse. Something you can take or leave alone. Consequently, some of the things you once thought were play are now really drudgery. Bowling leagues, coffee klatches, bridge nights, and even jogging. Though they began with play in mind, they may have turned into an obligation you can't or won't give up. You'd like to quit the softball team, but the girls are counting on you. You have to attend the neighborhood study group because, well, it's expected of you. Soon, play has become work.

To remedy that, look for new ways to play. Usually that means returning to basic, simple activities, perhaps even activities that are childish. The activities listed in the next chapter and section can be used. For starters, a hobby or special project can be play. Hobbies are often abandoned by adults when they enter the work/family bandwagon. Interestingly, that's when stress usually begins to become a problem. If you collected stamps in the sixth grade, dig out your old collection—it may rekindle interest and give you something to play with. If that doesn't suit you, try something on the creative side. Learn to dance. Grab a brush, canvas, and palette, and give painting a try. Or learn to play a musical instrument. The goal is not to become a world master but to divert your attention from the doldrums while having a little fun.

Expression of Feelings and Emotional Awareness

Emotional health and a zest for living are impossible unless we can acknowledge our feelings and learn how to express them appropriately and use them effectively. Unfortunately our culture does not respect emotions, and we are taught to hide, deny, or repress our feelings lest we "lose control" and "act irrationally."

This is particularly true in the business world, where the direct expression of feelings is usually discouraged, and where the ability to deal with feelings is much less valued than the capacity to handle ideas. Nevertheless, as behavioral scientists have noted, many of the most desirable traits in business—as well as personal life—are derived from emotions. These valuable qualities include creativity, motivation, loyalty, enthusiasm, and cooperation.

When feelings are stifled—whether at home or on the job—the results are poor. To begin with, the person harboring "unacceptable" emotions cannot function fully and freely, for precious energy must be wasted to maintain an inauthentic self, to create an "image," and to "play the game." Furthermore, if feelings are not shared and dealt with face-to-face, problems that have been "solved" by rational means don't stay solved for long—the underlying emotional conflict simply translates itself into other terms, erupting sooner or later into another crisis at work or home.

On the other hand, there is experimental evidence suggesting that if a person is allowed to express negative feelings to the individual who has aroused them, he or she will feel friendlier later than if the bad feelings are forced to remain "underground." If the expression of anger, anxiety, or frustration is not met with a counterattack or with an immediate attempt to introduce rationality, but is encouraged by the listener and received with understanding and acceptance ("You seem upset. What's troubling you? . . ." "I know how you feel."), then the upset person will be able to work through the negative feeling and arrive at a more objective assessment of the situation. The point is that "feelings press for discharge," and when they are denied they can become a barrier to closeness with others and to working rationally and harmoniously toward common goals.

The growing Re-evaluation Counseling (RC) movement is based upon the foregoing premise, which participants find to be borne out by experience. RC theory maintains that everyone is born with a great intellectual and emotional potential that gradually becomes blocked by an accumulation of distressing experiences that have not been worked through. When the pent-up fear, hurt, loss, anger, or embarrassment programmed in by these old distresses is released through adequate emotional discharge, the person is freed from rigid ways of acting and feeling and is able to act rationally and to be the flexible, loving, cooperative, intelligent and zestful being he or she was meant to be.

Handling Problems

Dealing with problems isn't peripheral to life, it's the essence of it, for whether we realize it or not, most human behavior consists of problem solving. Those who have the most success at understanding and solving problems independently or with the help of others have been found to share one characteristic: considerable confidence in and esteem for themselves and others. This kind of positive, facilitating attitude toward dealing with problems can be developed by jettisoning useless emotions, such as guilt, which shackles us to the past, or worry, which projects us into the imagined future. As psychologist Wayne Dyer has noted, neither of these all-too-common feelings changes anything; they can only rob us of the confidence and self-esteem we sorely need to tackle the problem and—equally harmful—distract us from the problem while siphoning off energy that should be directed into purposeful action.

Another tendency that undermines our ability to deal with problems is blaming. When we spend time and energy cursing fate or railing against people, circumstances, or even ourselves, we are simply expressing frustration. We are not correcting the problem. Indeed, by indulging in blame we are persuading ourselves that we are passive victims incapable of righting what's wrong.

I met a young sales representative who was like that. He blamed his company for sending him into such a nonproductive area. He blamed his customers for being too conservative. He blamed the economy for his dismal sales record. He even blamed his family for "holding him back." Since most of his energy was wrapped up in blaming, he accomplished very little. He convinced himself that he was powerless to overcome his problems and was willing to struggle along in an anemic fashion.

Guilt, worry, blame, and fear all promote procrastination, and are most likely to do so when we are confronted by a problem. To fight the tendency to avoid problems by taking refuge in delay, time management consultant Alan Lakein suggests strategies such as structuring your time and the things around you so you can't use your favorite escape routes, such as saying to yourself, "I'm wasting my time" whenever you find yourself dodging a problem that needs attention. Possibility thinker Robert Schuller's technique is to make a habit of asking yourself, "What is your biggest problem and what have you done about it today?" Another approach to handling procrastination linked to stress is to train yourself to be more of a stress-seeker and to view problems as challenges.

Some interesting studies performed by Susan C. Kobasa and Salvatore R. Maddi, both psychologists at the University of Chicago, indicate that stress can be a positive element for some people. They contend that stress-resistant people have a specific set of attitudes toward life that make up what is known as a "hardy personality." *Those attitudes are an openness to change, a feeling of involvement in whatever they are doing, and a sense of control over events.* One of the studies showed that people who rated high in these attitudes had fewer stress-related illnesses than others. On the other hand, those who rated low in "hardiness" avoid their problems—distracting themselves by watching more TV, drinking too much, taking tranquilizers, and sleeping more. Instead of solving problems, they ignore them.

Steps in problem-solving as articulated by one successful executive are (1) to identify the problem, (2) to find the causes by investigation, (that is, by talking to all involved and asking Who-What-Where-How-and-When questions, then making comparisons and deductions), (3) to weigh the possible inferences, and (4) to decide on the best solution, which should be economical, efficient, fair, based on facts, and meet current needs but also anticipate future needs.

Self-Actualization

As human beings, we have a hierarchy of needs that must be met if we are to continue to live and to evolve as individuals. Our most basic need is the physiological one for food, air, and water and this will motivate us sufficiently in life-or-death situations, as will the next highest need, which is for security (protection from physical harm). As these requirements are met, we continue up the ladder, first seeking the fulfillment of social, or affiliative, needs, which represent the longing for acceptance by others, then striving to meet esteem, or ego needs, which involve recognition by others. At the very top of the hierarchy of needs most social scientists place self-actualization (sometimes called self-fulfillment). This has been variously defined as becoming one's best self, achieving self-recognition, making the decision to take responsibility for self-motivation, realizing one's potential, and continuing to grow and be creative.

The behavior characterizing self-actualizing people stands in sharp contrast to the self-destructive activities engaged in by those who have not been able to satisfy and transcend their more basic needs. Through interviews with selected subjects, psychologist Abraham Maslow found self-actualizers to be totally unique in the expression of their varied selves, yet alike in being authentic, involved in a cause outside themselves that makes the work-joy dichotomy disappear, and in devoting their lives to a search for ultimate values with which they identify themselves, such as truth, goodness, beauty, justice, order, aliveness, and playfulness.

Carl R. Rogers has described the "fully functioning person" as one who (1) is in flow, in the process of changing his/her self and personality, (2) is open to all of his/her experience, with more of his/her life available as a resource, (3) is experiencing in the present rather than being bound rigidly to the past,

(4) trusts his/her total being to select the most appropriate behavior and is learning to be "the passenger, not the driver" in the realization that the total organism may be wiser than its conscious awareness, (5) is creative because he/she is open to the world and trust his or her own ability to form new relationships with the world, and (6) lives a life of great richness of feeling because of an underlying self-confidence.

Maslow claims all of us have the impulse toward self-fulfillment, but most of us never make it because we fear our highest possibilities—a fact revealed by our mixed feelings toward great people. Society itself may be encouraging us to remain inhibited and self-divided. Rogers has come to believe that "individuals are culturally conditioned, rewarded, reinforced for behaviors that are in fact perversions of the natural directions of the unitary actualizing tendency."

Our task, then, is to give up only as much as we must to routine and tedium and to strike out on a unique path of lifelong learning which may, as Buckmister Fuller has suggested, involve the "self-administered unlearning of most of what we've been taught in school." We can hasten our progress toward self-actualization by (1) allowing ourselves to experience life fully, without self-consciousness or self-awareness, (2) making choices based on growth (progression) rather than fear (regression), (3) listening to our inner totality—The Self—rather than to the introjected voices of parents or other authority figures, (4) being honest when we are in doubt, (5) following our own tastes, (6) preparing ourselves to do well what we want to do, (7) seeking and surrendering to peak experiences, in which we transcend ourselves and experience moments of self-realization, and (8) identifying our defenses and finding the courage to give them up and to invest the people, events, and objects around us with symbolic and eternal value.

It's not going to be easy, this business of fighting back from a lifestyle based on almost total vulnerability to stress. There will be setbacks along the way, apparent failures. At times, you will be tempted to give up. I know that I face times like that occasionally, and usually they occur just when I think I've got things under control. So I'd like to share some thoughts with you that have helped me deal with those setbacks. I would like to claim them as my own kernels of truth, but the credit goes to Hans Selye:

1. Regardless of how much you want to be loved, it's useless to try and befriend someone who continuously rejects you.
2. Face the fact that there is no such thing as perfection. Your highest goal is to be the best *you* can be.

3. Returning to a more simple lifestyle can add more pleasure to life than all that wealth and extravagance you've been struggling to obtain.
4. Before you waste a lot of energy trying to fight your way out of a situation, ask yourself if it's really worth fighting for.
5. Focus only on what is pleasant in your life, forgetting anything painful or ugly.
6. When you face your most difficult hour, try to recall and dwell on a past success. A sense of frustration can totally immobilize you. You can avoid that by concentrating on even the slightest bright spot in your past.
7. Never try to detour from unpleasant tasks. Face them as soon as possible so that you can move on to more enjoyable things.
8. There are no pat answers or special formulas for success that will fit everyone. Choose from a wide variety of advice only those things that fit your own unique personality.

If you follow the suggestions in this chapter, you will NOT eliminate stress from your life. Stress is here to stay. However, applying these ideas to your life wherever they are relevant and possible will bring you a long way toward dealing with the stress that has sapped so much of your energy.

CHAPTER 8
The Three Rs

By now you have an idea of what stress is doing to your energy levels. You also have some ideas on how to deal with them. Here I want to give you some important extra helps—the three Rs: Relaxation, Recreation, and Rest. It is important to note that I use recreation in the true sense of the word: activities that recreate with a sense of newness and vitality.

You can't run from stress. You must face it head-on. You want to turn stress into positive energy. I'm convinced that one reason why so many people do not enjoy life is that they expend too much energy running from it, trying to avoid it. In this chapter you will discover some techniques and responses to stress that enable you to really live rather than merely exist.

You will recall that your body's first response to stress is alarm. That's good. It gets you going—really pumped up to do the job. Then, if the stress continues, your body gears itself for the battle. Again, that is natural and necessary. Your body is tapping its energy supply. The problems start when you don't give your body a chance to recover through some form of rest. It is at this point that you must intervene and take measures to master further stress.

Relaxation and Recreation: Their True Value

Free-lance financier Harry Browne has suggested that "success is more often achieved by individuals who found ways of enjoying themselves while in the process of getting where they wanted to go." If this is true, it may be because relaxation is the first and last term of creativity, for the most original ideas and insights tend to arise not in the midst of intense concentration but in moments of apparent idleness when the conscious mind is off-guard.

Such utility aside, the development of impersonal interests is important, if only because favorite physical or mental pursuits can provide a resource and a respite at times when our central concerns in life are going badly. Bertrand Russell found an abundant appreciation of life to be a positive good all by itself, declaring, "The secret of happiness is this: let your interests be as wide as possible, and let your reactions to the things and persons that interest you be as far as possible friendly rather than hostile."

But how do these friendly, impersonal interests get translated into true pleasure—that is, into the kind that is restorative? Drama critic Walter Kerr has written perceptively on this subject. As he suggests, fun doesn't yield to command but only to surrender. That is, the more we want or expect to have a good time, the less likely we are to have one—a phenomenon that applies to social events, sexual experiences, everything. It is necessary, says Kerr, to "quiet the will to please the mind"—to hold the self in abeyance and cultivate "a relaxed grip," a state of readiness that is *not* acquisitive. The paradox is that only by bringing ourselves to a willingness to let go can we firmly grasp the pleasure we so desire. The problem, Kerr maintains, is that "as twentieth-century adults we have become compulsive users," and have lost the ability to contemplate experiences, things, and people—that is, to view them attentively in an appreciative and relaxed, but nonacquisitive way. A direct contradiction to the way most Americans live.

Contemplation and the restorative pleasure it makes possible are also being threatened by the frantic pace of modern life, which keeps us so busy and distracted that we don't have time to contemplate even fragments of our experience, let alone the whole of our lives. The way back to this profound kind of recreation seems to lie in undoing the conditioning that our industrialized society has imposed on us—we must once again learn to value doing things, instead of getting them, and the insights that we can create for ourselves rather than the things and experiences we can buy.

Relaxation

We often misinterpret what type of "rest" our bodies need. After a grueling day at the office we reward ourselves by flopping down on the couch to rest and recover from our stress-filled day, when what your body really might need is physical activity. Or, you pour yourself a drink when a chat with your spouse would be better for both of you. As you will see from some of the stress management techniques discussed in this chapter, you need to reassess traditional methods of relaxing, i.e., sleep, rest, watching TV. Often, those only postpone the problem.

The first group of techniques here confront your stress via relaxation. They allow you to focus on the causes of stress and the resulting physical, mental, or emotional strain. Not all of them will work for you, but it will be helpful to try each exercise at least once before you pass judgment. Think of this section as a catalogue of techniques that are available for you. Some you may not need. Some may not work for you, yet they do wonders for the other guy. By becoming familiar with each of them you will be better equipped to turn stress into energy.

Body Scanning

This may sound exotic, but it isn't. It's a simple technique to become more aware of your body. Lie down on the floor and close your eyes. Starting with your toes, think your way up your body asking yourself, "Where do I feel tension?" If you discover your jaw muscles are tight, exaggerate them slightly by tightening them more. Remind yourself that this takes effort and if continued over a long period of time you will become exhausted. Then relax those muscles and move on to the next source of tension. This activity need not take more than five minutes. Try doing it just before you leave for work and again before going to bed.

Progressive Relaxation

This technique, and a book by the same name, was developed by Dr. Edmund Jacobson in the early 1900s. It is based on the premise that the body responds to anxiety-provoking thoughts with muscle tension and that deep muscle relaxation counters the effects of that tension. This has been found to be especially helpful in the treatment of anxiety, insomnia, depression, fatigue, high blood pressure, and neck and back pain.

Repeat the following procedures at least once, tensing each muscle group from 5 to 7 seconds and then relaxing from 20 to 30 seconds. Focus on the contrast between the sensations of tension and relaxation.

1. Curl both fists, tightening biceps and forearms. Relax.
2. Wrinkle up forehead. At the same time, press your head as far back as possible, roll it clockwise in a complete circle. Reverse. Now wrinkle up the muscles in your face by frowning, squinting, pursing your lips,

pressing your tongue against the roof of your mouth, and hunching your shoulders. Relax.

3. Arch back as you take a deep breath into the chest. Hold. Relax. Take a deep breath, pressing out the stomach. Hold. Relax.

4. Pull feet and toes back toward face, tightening shins. Hold. Relax. Curl toes while simultaneously tightening calves, thighs, and buttocks. Hold. Relax.

Make sure in the relaxation stage the muscle group is totally relaxed. When you think the muscles are completely relaxed, tell yourself to relax just a little bit more. Also, don't overly tighten the muscles when you are tensing, as it could cause a cramp.

This technique will take some practice at first. Eventually, however, it will be possible to relax your entire body in just a few moments. It's a great one for desk-sitters and can be performed almost anywhere.

Meditation

Meditation may take many forms, but regardless of how you meditate, it affects your body and mind and gives you energy in many different ways. Meditators state that 20 minutes of their activity is equivalent to the boost you expect to receive from a cup or two of coffee. Scientists tell us that the reason for this lift is that meditation causes a significant drop in metabolism. This drop is similar to several hours of sleeping—yet in meditation the drop is achieved in a matter of minutes. Heart rate and breathing also slow down while anxiety decreases.

Research also suggests that meditators learn how to handle their stress better. A study reported in the February 1976 issue of *Psychology Today* in the article, "Meditation Helps Break the Stress Spiral," by David Golman, illustrates this point. The experimenters selected two groups of people to watch a highly stressful film—accidents in a woodworking shop. One group consisted of experienced meditators while the other group of people wanted to learn meditation but had not yet tried it.

The researchers divided these people into two subgroups. Twenty minutes before the showing of the film the meditating people were told to either meditate or simply relax. One-half of the meditators relaxed for 20 minutes and the other half of the meditators meditated for 20 minutes. The other group of subjects was split in a similar manner. The first group was told to relax while the second group was taught a meditation technique in 20 minutes.

The results of the study were revealing. Those who had meditated (experienced and nonexperienced) had more signs of alarm just before an accident occurred on the screen. They had higher heart rates, more sweating, and so forth. Interestingly, they returned to normal more quickly afterwards, which indicates that their bodies were handling the stress quite well. The response to stress was true of all meditators—the novices included. Even the meditators who relaxed responded similarly. The researchers came to the inescapable conclusion that meditation apparently had immediate and long-term effects on your body. It had long-term effects since the experienced meditators who simply relaxed also handled the stressful viewing quite well. Meditation helps people cope better with stress.

There are many kinds of meditation. I'll simply include here a discussion on transcendental meditation and the Relaxation Response.

Transcendental Meditation (TM)

In TM there is first a ceremony in which each meditator receives his personal secret mantra as he kneels before a picture of a guru. As he is doing this his instructor chants in Sanskrit. The mantra is supposedly chosen for its relationship to the person's nervous system. These mystical aspects make some people feel uncomfortable with TM for they consider it a violation of their own faith. Regardless, the technique does seem to work in helping people relax and refill them with energy. Here's the TM technique:

1. If you have no guru to prescribe a mantra, select one that suits you. A mantra is a syllable, word, or name that is repeated many times as you free your mind of thoughts. Typical Eastern mantras are "OM" (I am) and "SO-HAM" (I am he) or "SA-HAM" (I am she).
2. Center yourself in a quiet place by either sitting in a chair, kneeling on the floor, or sitting cross-legged in a modified "Lotus position."
3. Pay special attention to relaxing your chest and throat.
4. Chant your mantra aloud. Let your mantra find its own rhythm as the sound of your voice fills you and makes you relax.
5. After about 5 minutes of chanting your mantra aloud, shift to whispering it. As you do so, relax deeper and deeper, flowing with the rhythm of the sound.
6. Chant 15 minutes a day, five to seven days a week for two weeks, at which time you may wish to increase the length of the sessions to 30 minutes. Try this form of meditation for about a month before deciding whether you will continue it or cease it.

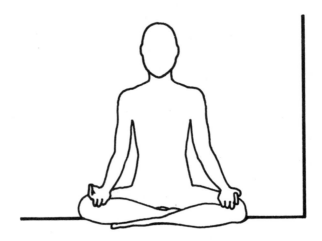

Illus. 8-1   The Lotus Position

As I said, some people have difficulty with some of these esoteric techniques. Consequently, the Relaxation Response and mental relaxation may be more to their liking.

Relaxation Response

Relaxation Response is a technique set forth by Dr. Herbert Benson, a Harvard cardiologist. After studying various ways of relaxing he found that meditation, yoga, praying, and similar kinds of activities elicited relaxation on the part of the participant and was probably energizing. Benson outlined a simple way of helping to soothe your body during stress. He suggests that you engage in the following Relaxation Response type of activity twice a day—early morning and in the evening. According to the cardiologist, you should begin your daily "destressing" with these suggestions:

1. Sit quietly in a comfortable position.
2. Close your eyes.
3. Deeply relax all your muscles, beginning at your feet and progressing up to your face. Keep them relaxed.
4. Breathe through your nose. Become aware of your breathing. As you breathe out say the word, "ONE," silently to yourself. For example, breathe IN . . . OUT, "ONE"; IN . . . OUT, "ONE"; and so on. Breathe easily and naturally.
5. Continue for 10 to 20 minutes. You may open your eyes to check the

time, but do not use an alarm. When you finish, sit quietly for several minutes, at first with your eyes closed and later with your eyes open. For a few minutes, do not stand up.

6. Do not worry about whether you are successful in achieving a deep level of relaxation. Maintain a passive attitude and permit relaxation to occur at its own pace. While distracting thoughts occur, try to ignore them by not dwelling upon them and return to repeating "ONE." With practice, the response should come with little effort. Practice the technique once or twice daily, but not within two hours after any meal, since the digestive processes seem to interfere with the elicitation of the Relaxation Response.

Imagining

As a youngster, you probably escaped the boredom of numerous situations by turning on your imaginative powers. Immediately, you left the stifling lecture period and joined King Arthur at the Round Table. By occasionally engaging in this same activity, you can treat yourself to some bright spots in what might be a stress-filled day.

There are no special rules to follow when you use your imagination to create relaxation and relief from stress. Whenever you sense a tenseness invading your body, close your eyes and try to imagine something especially pleasant: wading in a cool mountain stream, walking along a mountain trail, seeing a calm, blue sky, or gliding through the air in a rope swing. Always try to imagine yourself in a distant setting, away from your daily routine. Mentally plan the "ideal" getaway vacation.

After imagining for three to four minutes, open your eyes, change your position, stretch, and resume what you were doing. One caution: don't become a constant daydreamer. A few, brief sessions each day will give you a sense of heightened energy and emotional well-being. Spending more than five to ten minutes several times a day at this may cost you your job—thus more stress and less energy!

Breathing Exercises

Everyone knows how to breathe. Yet paying attention to different types of breathing can help restore energy lost through stress. Try the following techniques occasionally for a lift.

Deep Breathing

Lie down on the floor with your knees slightly bent, one hand on your abdomen, the other on your chest. Inhale deeply through your nose, trying to control your breathing with your abdomen. Your chest should move only a little. Smile slightly, exhaling through your mouth, making a quiet, relaxing sound like the wind as you gently release your breath. Continue for three to ten minutes.

Sighing

Sighs and yawns are signs that your body needs more energy-rich oxygen. A sigh provides you with a rush of air and helps to reduce tension. Simply take a deep breath and sigh deeply, letting out a sound of relief as the air leaves your lungs. (Whew!) Don't rush it and don't think about inhaling. Just let the air come in naturally. Repeat this six to eight times whenever you feel the need for it.

The Windmill Breath

Stand up with your arms stretched out at your sides. Take a deep breath and as you exhale slowly, swing your arms alternately like a windmill. Repeat two or three times. This is especially helpful if you have been bent over your work for several hours and are feeling tense. You will return to your work feeling more alert and alive.

Relaxation Throughout the Day

The mental relaxation drill mentioned earlier is a helpful "tool" to use occasionally to provide relief from stress. In addition to that, you need to program relaxing activities into your day. Choose anything that takes your mind off the hustle and bustle of everyday life and produces a pleasant feeling. Reading a book, enjoying a quiet talk with your spouse, working in the garden, helping one of your kids put together a model airplane, or listening to music. It is important that each day you experience this type of pleasant activity. It is essential in combating physical fatigue. If your loss of energy is due to extreme physical exertion, going out to run or walk may make you even more tired. Spending a few minutes genuinely relaxing can restore that lost energy and enable you to finish the day on an upbeat note.

Sometimes people equate relaxation with sitting or lying down. Often, that may be the case. Spending a few minutes with your feet elevated and a pillow under your head can be revitalizing. But don't limit yourself to that. Experiment with different activities to see what works best in taking your mind off your problems. If you work with your head all day, you may find a hobby that requires some manual skills is just the thing. If your job requires a lot of physical labor, reading, word games, writing, or learning something new might offer more relaxation for you. Find an activity that is best for you, then allow yourself time on a regular basis to enjoy that activity. Suffice it to say here that selected yoga postures and breathing may help you relax and therefore build your energy.

Recreation

In addition to contemplation, there are more active forms of recreation that are restorative. Most thoughtful people agree, however, that the kind of fun that renews and truly recreates us doesn't come from overstimulation. As pointed out in Chapter 5, overstimulation of any kind is exhausting and makes us "insensitive to the pleasures of ordinary living."

Just what kinds of activities meet the requirement of being restorative without being exhausting? Which ones give us more than they (or the world) take away? Bertrand Russell himself favored long nature walks and ocean swims, for he believed pursuits that bring mankind into contact with the life of the Earth are profoundly satisfying and make for lasting happiness even though their intensity may be less than that "of more exciting dissipations."

Noncompetitive activities such as jogging, or any other recreation meeting the criteria for a "positive addiction" (activities that build you up rather than tear you down—that are creative rather than destructive) are another route for self-renewal. Along these lines, a whole new approach to physical education has come into being, one that is person-centered instead of sports-centered. Promoted by the nonprofit New Games Foundation based in San Francisco, New Games' theory is built around cooperation and the participation of more people than can be included in the old-style competitive sports and games that favor the fittest and the feistiest. "Winning" in the New Games style of fun comes from competition that is self-motivated, not directed against others, and may involve participation in tying or untying a human knot, pushing an earth ball, or playing rotation volleyball.

Whatever the form of recreation we choose, it is important to remember that our psychological needs must be satisfied directly, through an active effort of our own, "and not by the substitution and distraction" and oblivion provided by escapist fare such as TV, drugs, and spectator sports. Passive entertainment makes us less alive. It is not renewing, just distracting. Real recreation can be had only by identifying our needs (which may, for example, be for physical, sensory, emotional, interpersonal, intellectual, social-political, creative-aesthetic, or spiritual experience) and seeking out the personal and community resources appropriate to satisfying them.

Below are some recreational physical activities that help to give us mastery over stress. They help build fitness, reduce tension, make us feel good about ourselves, and energize our bodies.

Running and Other Aerobic Activities

I mention running first because I think it should have high priority. It also is the activity that has had the most research conducted about it. Some physiologists and psychiatrists have begun to advocate the use of running as therapy for stress-related problems such as the blues, depression, nervous tension, and fatigue. Thaddeus Kostrubala, M.D., a California psychiatrist, requires each of his patients to run a specified time and distance several times a week. He often runs with them, conducting his counseling "on the run." If he doesn't run, one of his running therapists does.

John Griest, M.D., a psychiatrist operating out of the University of Wisconsin in Madison, has used running as a very important part of a therapy program with depressed patients. He found that fatigue was a common symptom of depression and that the running helped depressed individuals alleviate that "tired overall feeling." I interviewed one of his patients, and here's what she had to say.

> I used to be tired all the time and do nothing but sit around the house after work. Since I started on the running program, I've got the energy to do anything I want. I have this feeling that there's nothing stopping me now.

Dr. Griest added that he believes running is effective in helping to manage the blues or mild depressions because:

1. Anything that is repetitive in nature, allows people to relax, and gives them a feeling of accomplishment seems to be helpful in reducing depression.
2. Running requires patience. Through running, the person learns that it takes time to make significant physical changes. An appreciation of the value of patience may reduce depression.
3. Runners learn, often dramatically, that they can change themselves for the better. They see that they are sufficiently in control of their lives to be able to improve their health, appearance, and self-image.
4. Running helps them to develop a feeling of accomplishment. Any time you experience a sense of success, you'll probably be pulled out of depression.

There's probably another reason as well. There's an old comedy routine about a doctor who steps on his patient's foot to make the patient forget about his headache. There's something of that in the relationship between running and depression. Runners are forced to notice new and significant body sensations, which distract them. People who run tend to focus on the reality of sore calves or other muscle groups and forget about the symptoms of depression.

But not all research has been done on running. Activities such as walking are just as effective. Dr. Herbert deVries, Ph.D., a noted exercise physiologist, has said that the best tranquilizer is a brisk, 15-minute walk. One of his studies demonstrated that a short walk can be as effective in treating nervous tension as a normal dosage of a tranquilizer.

The next chapter explains in detail what is meant by aerobic exercise and how extra exercise reduces stress and builds energy. I realize that sounds contradictory. The mother who teaches school all day, returns home to make dinner and tend to her children, often is fatigued from high levels of stress. The last thing she feels like doing is running around the block. Yet it is important to realize such stress produces mental and emotional fatigue. Lying down on the couch may not help. Your nervous and hormonal systems have been stimulated all day and are physically geared up for a battle. The best thing to do, under those circumstances, is to simulate the "battle" with sustained, physical activity such as walking, running, bicycling, swimming, and dancing.

Your program of physical activity may be as informal and unstructured as adding a 15-minute walk to your lunch hour. Or, it might be as vigorous as a 40-minute run every day. The following guidelines will help you use physical activity to reduce stress-induced fatigue:

1. Choose an activity you enjoy—just because running is "in" doesn't mean you will enjoy it. Walking is just as effective and often fits into your daily routine quite easily.
2. Think of each session as a reward rather than an obligation—sometimes the anticipation of a little exercise is part of the "magic" of reducing fatigue.
3. Don't overdo it—within ten minutes after your exercise session, you should feel refreshed and ready to resume your schedule. If you are unduly tired and physically uncomfortable for a half hour or more after exercising, you probably overexercised. Take it easy, especially in the early stages.
4. Enjoy the physical "you"—take pride in the fact that you've joined a unique group of people who use stress rather than allow themselves to

be abused by it. Remind yourself, perhaps with an air of justifiable smugness, that someone else is taking a Seconal to escape while you have opted for self-discipline and control.

5. Don't worry about the clock. No horse ever tried to make the 7 A.M. train unless he had a rider on his back. Exercise at a rate that seems best for you. Do not keep comparing yourself to some arbitrary standard. The best recreation is play.

Yoga

Yoga has been shown to be effective in reducing anxiety, muscle tension, and muscle aches. In Chapter 10 I'll review its benefits in length.

Rest and Sleep

Rest is very important. You cannot have good energy levels without it. You might compare your body to a machine or engine, for it can generate power. As with other engines, however, it needs rest to avoid a breakdown since your body wears out a little each day. Fortunately, proper rest keeps you from disintegrating too much, for during rest your mind and body recharge themselves.

The Benefits of Sleep

As you know, your body is in action constantly. Sometimes slow, sometimes fast, but it's always working. When you're wide awake, your body is stimulated to a great extent. You're mentally alert. You're physically aware of things around you. Your nervous system is always being bombarded by different kinds of stimuli. After a period of time both your body and your mind call for a rest. They tell you it's time to slow down. When that happens you start to feel tired. You become drowsy. Sleep is the only way out. Your sleep will prepare you for the next day's activities.

The revitalization that occurs during sleep happens because your nervous system is no longer stimulated as previously. Your heart rate slows down as does your breathing rate. Your body temperature and blood pressure drop. Almost everything in your body slows down. The stimuli for your five senses are reduced substantially. It is during this time that your body's "batteries" are recharged. When you awaken you should be completely refreshed. Ready to go.

Scientists feel that it's difficult to make up for sleep that is lost. While it's true that you may be able to get by on no sleep for one night and then get 16 hours the next, your body apparently does not work that way. In fact, some specialists feel that each time you fail to get an adequate amount of sleep you lose extra brain cells; cells that cannot be replaced. It seems better to try to get your proper allotment of sleep each night or day rather than to stay up late one night and then try to catch up the next.

REM and Non-REM Sleep

Scientists who have been studying the pattern of sleeping recently say that there are two kinds of sleep. One of these is called Rapid Eye Movements or REMs, during which you dream vividly. The other type of sleep is Non-REM, of which there are four stages.

First Stage: Here, you're just falling asleep. Your body functions are starting to slow down. But you can be awakened easily.

Second Stage: During this stage your eyes roll from side to side. Your sleep is deep. But when you awaken you do not recall having any dreams.

Third Stage: Your body really slows down in this stage. Blood pressure and pulse rates are very low, as is your temperature. Sleep is very deep and calm.

Fourth Stage: This is the period of deepest sleep. But it is brief. Nightmares and sleepwalking can occur during this stage.

After getting to the fourth stage, you then go back to stages three, two, one, and into REM sleep. During your sleep you move continually through these stages. As the night continues, the REM time gets longer and the Non-REM time shorter. REM sleep occurs about three to four times a night. Each occurrence lasts from five minutes to over an hour. Interestingly, as much as 50 percent of an infant's sleep is REM sleep. With an adult, about 20 percent is REM sleep.

The amount of REM sleep is very important, because the degree of restfulness of sleep is related to the amount of REM sleep. The more REM sleep, the more rest. Studies have been done where people were awakened each time they entered REM sleep. The result was extreme tiredness and abnormal behavior on the part of these subjects.

How Much Sleep Do' You Need?

Everyone needs sleep. Some need more, some less. Most young people need somewhere around 8 to 10 hours of sleep. Newborn babies may sleep as much as 20 hours or more a day. Mature adults usually find 7 hours or less is sufficient. But even in these ages there are differences. Thomas Edison is said to have slept only 3 to 4 hours a night. He did however have a cot in his laboratory and he catnapped whenever fatigue got the best of him.

Napping

Two well-known catnappers of the twentieth century are Dr. Michael DeBakey, the world famous heart specialist, and the late President John F. Kennedy. DeBakey is able to fall asleep very quickly. When traveling by air, he simply buckles himself into his seat on the plane and immediately drops into a deep sleep. President Kennedy was able to do the same thing. During a busy and pressure-packed day, he could fall asleep quickly. He would sit down, close his eyes, and fall asleep almost immediately. In five minutes he would awaken refreshed and ready to dive into the task at hand.

People like DeBakey, Kennedy, and Edison are exceptions. So are their jobs. The work world is set up on an eight-hour sleep schedule. Most people turn in somewhere between 9:00 P.M. and midnight and arise between 5:00 and 8:00 A.M. As a result, most people get their eight hours of sleep or so in one block of time.

Regardless, a proper amount of sleep is very important for everyone. But each person's requirements for sleep will vary. Some may need nine hours of sleep, some feel seven is enough. The key to understanding whether you are getting enough is that you should awaken spontaneously and refreshed.

Sleep Disorders

People who are depressed tend to sleep or want to rest a great deal. Other people find that they enjoy sleeping simply because it helps them to escape reality. They're upset with their lot in life and they use sleep as a security blanket. Eventually the depression becomes more and more complex, because, as people sleep, they start to get down on themselves, they feel lethargic, and they lose their fitness level. As a result their self-concept starts to slip and they feel even more depressed.

People who do not get enough sleep ofttimes lose energy and become quick-tempered. If you go for about two days without sleep you will lose your ability to concentrate. You may be able to force yourself to do some task for a short period of time, but lengthy tasks become impossible. You make many mistakes and are easily distracted. Three days without sleep only makes matters worse. You have a lot of difficulty thinking, seeing, and hearing. You may even suffer from hallucinations.

Insomnia

All people at one time or another have difficulty sleeping. Some people fall asleep rather quickly but awaken in the middle of the night. Some sleepwalk or talk in their sleep. The extent to which these disorders are serious depends upon how frequently they occur. The disorders are serious if they are disturbing to the sleeper or, I should say, nonsleeper.

Insomnia, however, is the inability to sleep. One out of every 20 people react this way. The problem is vicious. When a person goes to bed, tosses and turns and cannot sleep, he worries. He worries because he's not getting enough sleep so he stays awake even longer—sometimes the entire night. The next night when he falls into bed he's exhausted. But he's worried. Last night he didn't get enough sleep. So he worries about this and consequently loses even more sleep. The cycle progresses in this manner: worry, less sleep, more worry, less sleep, and so on. Worrying about the insomnia only makes matters worse.

To help themselves, some people use tranquilizers and barbiturates. But these drugs interfere with sleep. A number of researchers now have been able to explain why. Two of them are psychiatrists Raymond Greenburg and Chester Pearlman of the Veterans Administration Hospital in Jamaica Plains, Massachusetts. They report that people who take barbiturates or tranquilizers to get to sleep are dangerously altering their sleep patterns. These and other drugs make it impossible for the body to get to the most beneficial stage of sleep— the REM phase. During REM time we act out our frustrations, or sift through the day's experience, or indulge in wish fulfillment. So important are dreams as a safety valve that when we are deprived of REM time for one night, we will spend twice as much time dreaming the next night. And, if we deprive ourselves of dream time over a period of nights by taking drugs, we may show signs of disturbed, often neurotic, daytime behavior. Additionally, we usually wake up completely exhausted because the REM time was not sufficient to give us the deep sleep that is needed. The more REM sleep, the more rest.

There are ways of getting the rest you need without resorting to these kinds of medications. One of the best is a combination of exercise and relaxation. Frederick Baekland, M.D., D.M.Sc., of the State University of New York, Brooklyn, reported that people who follow a regular exercise program experience more healthful, invigorating sleep than those who don't exercise.

Baekland used 14 student volunteers, recording their brain wave patterns during sleep for one month. During this time, the students, all physically active, were not permitted to exercise. Near the end of the month of exercise deprivation the students were asked to fill out questionnaires concerning their experiences and feelings during the test period.

In studying the electroencephalogram (EEG) charts and completed questionnaires, Baekland found that the most striking change was that the REM density (period of light sleep with much dreaming) increased remarkably in the students deprived of exercise. These students also reported more frequent awakenings during the night, a decrease in appetite, increases in sexual tension and the need to be with others. The EEG also recorded a higher number of body movements in the students. Perhaps this was their subconscious attempt to make up for the exercise they had lost.

Baekland's experiment also proved that the students who exercised daily were able to enjoy more of the beneficial deep sleep than the students who did not exercise. Students following their regular fitness program tended to awaken refreshed, and did not develop any of the psychological difficulties experienced by those students deprived of activity.

The study shows that if we don't exercise properly we're just too wound up to benefit from a night's sleep. We drag ourselves from bed every morning, our nerves jangled, our eyes baggy. We face each day with a growl instead of a smile. Yet by combining a program of intermittent relaxation with a sensible daily exercise routine, each of us would soon find ourselves taking rapid steps to dreamland. An excellent approach is to modify the progressive relaxation technique described earlier in this chapter.

Most times insomnia occurs because of worry, tension, stress, and possibly other poor health habits. Here are some additional guidelines to help overcome insomnia.

1. Do not eat a heavy meal before going to bed.
2. Do not watch TV or read an exciting book before retiring.
3. Take a warm bath before retiring.
4. Drink a warm beverage just before bed.
5. Occupy yourself with a quiet hobby.
6. Take a leisurely walk before retiring.
7. Consciously try to relax the muscles of your body. Start with your feet and work your way up your body.
8. Try reading a very boring or dull book.
9. Get involved in a good overall aerobic fitness program.

The three Rs are basic to your energy needs. You can't go through life on hype. You need time to relax and recreate. You need time to recharge your batteries.

Your first Three Phase Plan follows. In this and the other plans, take the test to determine whether you should enter at Phase I, Phase II, or Phase III. Then, give the plans a chance. If you stay with a plan for two or three weeks, you will begin to notice positive changes in your energy levels.

A Three Phase Plan for Enjoying Life

The following test will give you a fairly objective indication of how much you enjoy life. From the scoring on this test plus a general idea of how much you think you enjoy life, you can determine at what level you should begin to fight back.

Enjoyment of Life Test*

Directions: For each question, check Yes or No. If you feel that you do not know the answer, or if it is one half yes and one half no, check both yes and no.

	Yes	No
1. Do people who know you well think you get upset easily?	___	___
2. Do people who know you well think you are stubborn?	___	___
3. Do people who know you well think you understand other people's points of view and accept them the way they are?	___	___
4. Do people who know you well think that when you get mad you get over it quickly?	___	___
5. Do people who know you well think you overcome problems easily?	___	___
6. Do people who know you well think you are reliable and responsible in meeting your financial obligations?	___	___
7. Do people who know you well think you have continued to mature and grow emotionally as you have gotten older?	___	___
8. Do you like being among people, sharing interest in activity, going out socially?	___	___
9. Do you think that changing your life in some way might make it easier to get well once you get sick?	___	___
10. Is it reasonably easy for you to get to know people and make friends?	___	___
11. Do you have good health?	___	___
12. Do you think you had a satisfying religious education?	___	___
13. Are you pleased when a friend is praised in your presence?	___	___
14. Can you be friendly and sociable with the opposite sex without any feeling of awkwardness and strain?	___	___
15. Do you think those close to you provide the emotional support you need?	___	___

*SOURCE: Dr. Donald L. Dudley and Elton Welke, "How to Live with Stress," *Forum International Journal of Human Relations*, November 1977, pp. 14–15.

Plan for Enjoying Life—Continued

	Yes	No
16. Can you take criticism and instruction in a good spirit?	___	___
17. Are you satisfied with your occupation?	___	___
18. Are you satisfied with your working conditions?	___	___
19. Is your income satisfactory?	___	___
20. Have you set goals for the future that satisfy you and are realistic?	___	___

Scoring: To score the test, give yourself +5 points for every Yes answer and −5 points for every No answer, except for questions #1 and 2. For these two questions, a No answer receives a +5 points and a Yes answer receives −5 points. Where you've answered Yes and No to an item you receive 0 points. Determine your total score. It will lie somewhere between −100 and +100.

80 to 100—You seem to enjoy life—enter at Phase 3.
40 to 80—You're not sure you really enjoy life—enter at Phase 2.
Negative score to 40—You do not find life enjoyable—enter at Phase 1.

Phase One—Identify the Sources of Stress in Your Life*

To help you more clearly understand some of the reasons why life may not be so enjoyable for you, check any of the following conditions that apply to you:

___ 1. Too many people to relate to.

___ 2. Frequent overtime and long hours.

___ 3. Egotistical fellow employees or supervisors.

___ 4. Excessive deadlines to meet.

___ 5. Excessive technical and repetitive work.

___ 6. Deluge of seemingly senseless paperwork.

___ 7. Fear of the consequences of making mistakes.

___ 8. Excessive noise.

___ 9. Extreme smells, sights, heat, and cold.

*Source: Adapted from Ron Clinton's stress inventory in *How to Prevent Burnout and Achieve Personal Well Being* (Detroit: Human Potential Pub., 1980).

Plan for Enjoying Life—Continued

_____10. Smoke and toxic substances in the air.

_____11. Feeling of incompetence.

_____12. Job seems meaningless and unchallenging.

_____13. Lack of true friends to share feelings with.

_____14. Current physical problems.

_____15. Failing marriage.

_____16. Poor money management resulting in excessive debt.

_____17. Long drive to and from work and rush hour traffic.

_____18. Overcommitment to clubs, organizations, church, etc.

_____19. Strained relationships with the children.

_____20. Not enough time for recreation and hobbies.

Additional Conditions

_____21.

_____22.

_____23.

_____24.

_____25.

Now go over the list above and select the three major sources of stress in your life:

1. _____

2. _____

3. _____

Phase Two—Attack One "Stress Target"

From the list of stress sources you selected in Phase One, select one as your "target" for one week. Plan an all-out attack on that target. Your plan will include the following components:

1. **Devise a realistic time schedule.** There are many ways to do this. One simple method is to use 3 × 5 index cards for each day of the week. On one side of the card, simply list your primary tasks and secondary tasks. On the other side, write down a time schedule for the day.

Plan for Enjoying Life—Continued

Example

Primary	
Staff meeting	
Bob—airport	
Timmie's concert	
Secondary	
Call L.A.	
Read new report	
Work on old accounts	

front

Monday	
6:30	Wake-up
7:15	Leave for work
8:30	Staff meeting
1:00	Call L.A. office
3:30	Meet Bob at airport
8:00	Timmie's concert

back

2. **Approach primary tasks with a positive attitude.** As you write down your primary tasks, think or concentrate on the good that will happen when you finish the task. For example:

Primary Task: Complete the refinishing job I started on the kitchen table and chairs.

Positive Results: 1. Family won't have to eat on TV trays scattered throughout the house.
2. Will be able to put my kitchen back in order.
3. Will give me a sense of pride and accomplishment.
4. Will give me time to enjoy something else.

3. **Take time to confide in someone.** This, perhaps, will be the most difficult, but could also help you the most. Select someone you can trust and make it a point to spend some time with that individual for the sole purpose of sharing your feelings and emotions.

4. **Take charge of your problems.** Write down one major problem you must face this week:

_____

Plan for Enjoying Life—Continued

Now list at least three ways of handling that problem. Do not include "ignoring it" as an option.

_____

_____

_____

Select what you think is the best option and apply that solution to the problem.

5. **Anticipate obstacles that may stop you.** Beat those obstacles to the punch. If you think about them ahead of time, you will already have an idea of how to get around them. Write down any obstacles that you think will stand in your way:

_____

_____

_____

6. **Meet those obstacles head on.** For any of the obstacles that you selected, write down how you plan to get around those obstacles:

_____

_____

_____

7. **Recognize your own personal value.** Begin or end each day by thinking about those things about you that make you proud of yourself. This can be done while commuting to work, jogging or walking, or lying in bed.

Phase Three—Make the Fight Enjoyable

In the first phase you got a handle on the cause of your stress. In Phase Two you began to fight back. In Phase Three you will continue the fight by adding other "stress targets" to your hit list. But now, you are beginning to master your problems. The fight is now becoming a challenge. Instead of looking at life as a series of problems to overcome, you view each day as a challenge and find excitement in trying to meet that challenge. Some things that will help you turn the fight into a challenge are included below:

Rest—If you ignore this element, you may not have enough energy to keep up with your enjoyable lifestyle.

1. Go to bed one half-hour earlier than normal. If you aren't tired enough to sleep, use the time to read, write letters, talk with your spouse, or listen to music.

Plan for Enjoying Life—Continued

2. If you are using a sleeping aid such as a barbituate or a tranquilizer, stop for at least a two-week trial period. If you have difficulty sleeping during that time, try some of these methods.

    A. Drink a cup of warm milk or herb tea one half-hour before retiring.
    B. Read something that is not related in any way to your work. Fiction is usually better for this than nonfiction.
    C. Exercise leisurely for 10 minutes just before going to bed.
    D. Take a hot bath before you retire.
    E. Practice a relaxation technique while lying in bed.
    F. Try falling asleep to soft music.
    G. Sip a half glass of wine 20 minutes before retiring. (Caution: if you are a regular moderate to heavy drinker, this will be of no help. Most alcoholics are plagued with insomnia.)
    H. Do not drink any coffee, tea, cola, or eat chocolate after noon.

Recreation—Put the play back into your life . . . even if it means being a kid again.

1. If you do not already do it, perform an aerobic activity (jogging, walking, swimming, etc.) for at least 20 minutes a day three times a week.

2. Once each week, participate in a noncompetitive physical activity with your family or friends. Suggested activities include:

Free-form wrestling and tumbling	Skiing (snow or water)
Imitate animal motions	Canoeing or sailing
Backyard obstacle course	Archery
Playground equipment play	Tree climbing
Dancing	Horseback riding
Hiking (on foot or bike)	Skating (ice or roller)
Sledding and tobogganing	Ping-Pong and badminton

Note: Traditional recreational activities like golf, bowling, softball, etc., are fine if a) competition does not become serious, b) a regular obligation does not turn it into a chore, c) relationships with family and/or friends do not play second fiddle to the activity.

Relaxation—Practice daily at least one of the relaxation techniques outlined in Chapter 8.

Here's a handy chart that may help you identify techniques for dealing with stress. As you can see, more than one stress reduction technique is available for most of the symptoms. Pick the one that seems to work best for you.

Plan for Enjoying Life—Continued

Stress Factors Affected by Relaxation, Recreation, and Rest Techniques

	Boredom	Anxiety	Blues	Depression	Anger	Tension	Fatigue	Insomnia	Muscle Twitches	High Blood Pressure	Muscle Ache Headache Backache
Aerobic Exercise	*	*	*		*		*	*		*	*
Breathing		*	*	*		*	*				
Body Scanning						*			*		*
Imagining		*				*			*		*
Mental Relaxation		*								*	
Progressive Relaxation		*	*	*		*	*	*	*	*	*
Relaxation Response		*	*	*	*		*	*		*	*
Relaxing	*		*								
Sleep		*					*			*	
Time Management		*	*	*	*		*				
Transcendental Meditation						*	*	*		*	*
Yoga & Yoga-Type Activities							*	*	*	*	*

SOURCE: Adapted from Martha Davis, Elizabeth R. Eshelman, and Matthew McKay, *The Relaxation and Stress Reduction Workbook* (Richmond, CA: New Harbinger Publications, 1980), pp. 14–15.

How to Use This Chart: From the list at the top of the chart, find the stress factor that pertains to you. Then look down that column and find the techniques marked with an asterisk that will help you cope with that factor.

ENJOYING FITNESS

CHAPTER 9
LSD and the O₂ High

I've been coming down hard on drugs all through this book, so you're probably surprised that now I'm recommending LSD. But I do recommend it. To me, LSD refers to Long Slow Distance. That's the best way to acquire the O₂ High.

This is not a lot of hocus-pocus I'm giving you. I really believe in getting high on O₂—oxygen. And the best way to get this type of "high" is through aerobic activities.

Aerobic Activity

Over a decade ago, Dr. Kenneth Cooper, author of *Aerobics*, began using the word that has since become a household term for people who exercise. That word is "aerobic." It means "with oxygen." It is my belief that participating in vigorous activities that use large amounts of oxygen (activities that make you huff and puff) will help you develop a boundless supply of energy. I feel it is the best type of energy-building exercise. To me, aerobic exercise is the foundation of any energy plan. I know this sounds strange, use energy to get energy. After all, that's the opposite of oil, gas, or nuclear energy. Believe me, though, it works with the body.

Let's take a close look at aerobic exercise. Just what do I mean when I toss that concept around? In my travels throughout the United States and Canada, I've noticed a rapid increase in the activity levels of most people. Practically everyone owns a double-knit jogging suit. Tennis courts are being built at a rapid rate, yet it's still difficult to find an empty court. Athletic facilities are in use almost 24 hours a day. Ditto for racquetball, handball, and squash courts. Ten years ago, you could mention the word Adidas and few would know that you were referring to an athletic shoe company. Now, at cocktail parties and church socials it is not uncommon to hear lively debate on the merits of a Brooks RT-1 over a New Balance 420. It seems as if everyone is climbing aboard the fitness wagon.

And that's good! It's good, except for one thing. Most of the activities that people choose are not aerobic. They are good, wholesome, fun activities, but they do little to increase your innate supply of energy. If you are concerned with getting more energy out of each minute, you need to spend some time each or every other day with one of the big four: running, walking, swimming, or cycling. Other energy-building activities are cross-country skiing and ice or roller skating. These are activities which can be done slowly, for a long period of time.

As you can see, these activities all have something in common. They are rhythmical, sustained, and you pay as you go. They offer no pause for station identification. They are not too strenuous, which means you can keep at them for 20 minutes to an hour. You never reach a point of total exhaustion, though your pulse increases, your breathing is heavier, and you may sweat a bit. That's what aerobic exercise is all about. Any activity that demands a steady use of oxygen for at least 20 minutes is considered aerobic.

As a contrast, most sports and leisure-time activities do not meet those requirements. They are either too hard or too easy. Take, for example, tennis. I really enjoy a game of tennis, even though I'm not very good. But I seldom get a real workout from a tennis game. Occasionally, my opponent gets me racing back and forth trying to return his shot. When that happens I really have to work. But it never lasts very long. A minute at the most. By then, I usually hit the ball into the net or miss altogether. Either way, we both get close to a minute's rest. We retrieve balls. Check equipment. Chat. Walk back to our positions. Then wait some more while I double-fault. Even if I play several games over an hour or so, I seldom have to breathe hard for more than five minutes at a time. Consequently, my activity is not aerobic.

Another popular activity is weight lifting. Every spa and fitness center worth its price of admission has a shiny array of weights and weight machines. Yet this activity does not qualify as aerobic because it's too hard. Most lifting is done in sets. That is, the lifter will pump the iron seven to ten times, then rest. You *have* to rest or you'd simply drop. That's because weight lifting places a heavy demand on selected muscles, not your whole body. After 30 to 40 seconds, your exercising muscles are taxed beyond belief. Try as you may to go beyond that length of time, your body simply says no. Before lifting again, you must rest, during which time your muscles recover. When lifting, your pulse rate increases, partly because your body's muscles need more oxygen and partly because the strain of lifting causes your blood pressure to increase markedly. It is impossible to steadily lift weights for 20 to 30 minutes. Your muscles would not permit you to do it.

Don't get me wrong. These are fine activities and it's encouraging to see more and more people choosing an active way of life over a more sedentary lifestyle. I love to play handball and tennis and I lift weights regularly. These activities build some energy. For example, the tennis and handball allow me to get the competitive urges out of me. They also help me release some anger. Whacking a ball hard helps me release a lot of tension and frustration in a socially acceptable way.

My weight-training conditions different muscles. Well-toned muscles make my body look better. If my body looks better, that gives me a psychological lift. I feel good about the way I look. Also, that lift, believe it or not, gives me energy.

Additionally, vigorous exercise of any type will cause a temporary lift because of possible biochemical changes. But more on that later in this chapter.

To some people, the concept of getting more energy from exercise is hard to grasp. Their reasoning seems to make sense: "If I go out and walk or play tennis for a half-hour, I'll be dead tired for the rest of the day." They argue that running, walking, swimming, tennis, and so forth make you dog tired afterwards.

Actually, the reverse is true. Exercise immediately produces an increase in energy. If you doubt me, try this experiment: some evening just before you normally retire, get in a good bout of healthy exercise. For most, a fast, vigorous walk will do. Go to the point where, after 30 minutes, you are pleasantly tired. Come home and immediately try to sleep. I guarantee you that you'll be *wide awake* for at least two hours. Why that happens has not been definitely answered, but good theories abound. The late Paul Dudley White, dean of American cardiologists, said, "The brain . . . needs to be well fed with oxygen and other chemicals and its waste products removed. Only the blood can do that. For its optimal function, therefore, the brain must have a good fresh supply which is delivered by a good heart and good blood vessels which should be kept in good condition."

Dr. A. H. Ishmail at Purdue University said essentially the same thing: exercise can produce physiological and biochemical changes, such as improved circulation which brings more oxygen to the brain. Better circulation means that the brain is getting greater amounts of glucose, a substance vital to its nutrition.

The National Institute of Health has speculated that there is an increase in the number or amount of neurotransmitters that give a person a psychological lift or an "awake" feeling. They are conducting experiments to investigate these and other biochemical changes that occur in the brain when a person is exercising.

I want to emphasize that nonaerobic activities may not give you energy in the same way as aerobic activities. They may even contribute to the energy drain that's been bothering you, simply because you're not in shape to play the sport. If the tennis match leaves you feeling sore, worn out, and tired the next day, it's because you're simply not in adequate condition to play it.

What special qualities of aerobic exercise make it the energy builder it is? There are many, including an increase in oxygen uptake, reduction in body fat, stress transfer, anger and anxiety abatement, a lift out of depression, and increased productivity and creativity.

Oxygen Uptake

I told you earlier that aerobics meant "with oxygen." As you know, human life depends upon oxygen. Without it we die. Similarly, with reduced amounts of it we are slowed down. When the human body becomes inefficient in transporting oxygen to various parts of the body, a lack of energy occurs.

Let's say you go visit a friend who lives in Mexico City. You're now at an altitude of 7,500 feet plus. The amount of oxygen in the air is reduced by about 40 percent. While visiting there you try to function at your usual level of activity. This might include a vigorous walk, a run, or simply cleaning the house. Very quickly you discover you are unable to maintain your normal pace for very long, because you're not getting as much oxygen as you normally get. Most likely, out of frustration, you will have to sit down and rest. My point? If your body does not obtain and use oxygen efficiently, no matter what the cause, you are forced to slow down. Your energy level drops off. You can't get enough oxygen.

Oxygen permits your muscles to contract, your brain to think, and your digestive system to digest. Of course, most of us are able to take in enough oxygen to "get through" our day. But unless we have good aerobic capacity, our efficiency in handling oxygen is not what it should be.

Proper amounts of oxygen permit your cells and tissues to work in an efficient manner. Oxygen is delivered to your tissues by means of your heart, blood, and blood vessels. When you are fit, your circulatory system becomes more efficient. Regular aerobic exercise may:

1. Increase the number and size of your blood vessels for better and more efficient circulation.
2. Increase the elasticity of the blood vessels, thereby permitting more blood to be circulated.
3. Increase the efficiency of exercising muscles and blood circulation so that muscles and blood are better able to pick up, carry, and use oxygen.
4. Increase the efficiency of the heart, making it able to pump more blood with fewer beats.
5. Increase the number of red blood cells so that more oxygen can be carried throughout your body.

These five things, plus some other complicated biochemical changes over a period of weeks and months, permit your body to improve its ability to pick up, deliver, and use oxygen. The result is more oxygen available to the tissues. And more oxygen to the tissues means more energy. It's as though you have been recycled from being a gas guzzler of the 60s and early 70s to being a fuel-efficient automobile of the 80s. You get more mileage from the same amount of energy.

A report by Dr. Roy J. Shephard, of the University of Toronto, Department of Physiological Hygiene, notes that an individual's aerobic fitness capacity typically declines with age. By 60, many men and most women are unable to work an eight-hour day without suffering from fatigue. But, says Dr. Shephard, "through the use of an appropriate training program [aerobic exercise], it is possible to improve working capacity by at least 15 or 20 percent." Working capacity, of course, has to do with endurance and stamina. With conditioning comes a greater capacity to get things done. You are able to do more before feeling fatigued. You have more "pep."

Spending 20 minutes or more on aerobic activity at least three days a week will give you more bounce to the ounce and more pep to the step. Or, to look at it another way, aerobic exercise recharges your body, much like a car battery is constantly recharged while the engine is running. Aerobic exercise is the prerequisite to an exciting life of increased energy. True energy begins with aerobic fitness.

Reduction of Body Fat

One of the most obvious reasons for lack of energy is obesity. Although I discuss this more in Chapters 13 and 14, I think it is important to touch a few highlights here. Many Americans simply have to work too hard because they carry around excess body fat. From the ages of 20 to 50, the average

American gains between 1 to 2 pounds of fat a year. Typically, we are fatter than the citizens of any other nation. It is not unusual for a middle-aged man or woman to be 20 to 30 pounds overfat. This extra fat robs you of energy.

Consider this: A bag of groceries weighs about 15 pounds. That's really not too heavy, but if for some reason you had to carry that bag any further than from the market to the car, you would get fatigued. Your arms would begin to tire. Your back would get sore. You would breathe harder carrying the load. Within a very short distance, you would run out of energy and either have to sit down and rest, or set the bag down.

That's just a crude illustration of how excess body weight drains us of our energy. Most people are no more than 10 to 15 pounds overfat, and yet that additional weight is enough to leave them feeling tired and run down. Instead of being able to "set the package down" and take a little rest, the overfat are forced to carry the weight all of their waking hours, upstairs and down, at the office, at the shop, at home. They trudge drearily through life with what could literally be described as excess baggage. No wonder we run out of energy so quickly—and avoid activity.

It doesn't have to be that way. If aerobic exercise did nothing else, the benefits from fat loss would be enough to give you noticeable extra energy, energy to help you enjoy more of each minute, and give you an extra hour or two of "fun time" after you get home from work. This energy can make your day at the office or plant more productive, and it comes from not having to carry around extra fat.

Extra fat is super if you are forced to eke out an existence on some desert island or country where starvation is rampant. But in those situations, survival is the crucial issue. In modern times, excess fat is really useless, because it is nonproductive tissue. It provides little benefit and makes your heart, lungs, muscles, bones, and other systems work harder. In other words, it wastes energy, gives you early fatigue, and makes you lethargic before your day is through.

If you are still having trouble with this concept, try this: Get a knapsack and put 15 to 20 pounds of books in it. Strap the pack on your back and carry it around for several hours. Then take it off. Notice how light you feel? How your step has a bounce to it? While you don't lose 15 to 20 pounds that quickly, the effect is the same. Once you shed the burden of extra fat, you will be able to work longer, play harder, and enjoy more of what life has to offer.

Aerobic exercise is the best way to reduce energy-wasting fat. To lose fat, you simply make sure you use more calories than you eat. That's simple enough. And, you have two ways to do this: diet or exercise. Dieting works, sometimes. But eventually the fat comes back because the regimen of a strict diet is too difficult for most humans. That's because we must eat to live. In addition, most diets rob you of your energy. Bill, a friend of mine, lost a great deal of weight by dieting. Then he quit his diet and gained it all back. When I asked him why, he responded, "I was constantly tired and hungry." That's no way to live. Yet recent statistics suggest that Americans spend over $10 billion a year trying to lose weight. On the average we go on 2½ diets per year in our quest to lose weight. Obviously, it must not be working. Additionally, researchers say that when you diet to lose weight you lose bone, muscle, and organ tissue as well as fat. And while those lost pounds may look good on the scale, they rob you of vital energy. Muscles give you go power! Your organs (brain included) need the proper number of cells to give you optimum energy. But fat robs you of it all.

A more sensible way to drop that unwanted load of fat without losing bone, muscle, and organ tissue is to burn off those extra calories through aerobic exercise. Any activity will do. Mopping the floor, or mowing the lawn. Going this route takes a real chunk of time. However, exercise that's aerobic in nature removes the fat quicker and more regularly. Why? By spending a half-hour a day, four to five days per week in an activity like bicycling, you will lose from 1,400 to 1,750 calories per week. Since 3,500 calories roughly equals one pound, in ten days you'll have dropped a pound. In just under three weeks, two pounds. Keep it up for six months and you will have dropped ten pounds. And that's with absolutely no change in your eating habits! You can have your cake, eat it too, and still lose fat, just from a half-hour of pleasurable bicycling, four to five times a week. If you want to lose it faster, you increase the time you spend doing it. Also, you can split that half-hour up any way you like. Do it all at once, or ride ten minutes before work, during your lunch break, and after work. Build it into your regular activities. It's that simple.

Exercise has been shown to have a pervasive effect on your emotional and mental health as well. By proven ways (and ways yet to be discovered), exercise is able to increase your energy level substantially. These include transfer of stress, anger, anxiety abatement, lifting of depression, and improved creativity and confidence.

Stress Transfer

I'm sure you've heard people say: "This job gives me a headache," or "I'm so mad my blood is boiling." As you know, these statements are quite correct. Frustrations, anger, hostilities, and headaches can give us high blood pressure and other energy-robbing diseases. You also know that a change in your activity can help you master those feelings. In a previous chapter we talked about relaxation techniques that would be helpful in managing stress. We learned from Dr. Hans Selye that "Stress on one system helps to relax the other." I want to show you here how exercise, specifically aerobic exercise, can give you mental and emotional energy.

A study conducted by Drs. John Boyer, M.D., and Fred Kasch, Ph.D., on 23 middle-age men with high blood pressure and 23 men with normal blood pressure demonstrated the effectiveness of six months of exercise on blood pressure. (High blood pressure robs people of personal energy.) The test subjects' routine consisted of 15 to 20 minutes of warm-up exercises, followed by walking and jogging. All of these men had been inactive before the program, and no attempt was made to alter their diet. At the end of the six months, there were significant reductions in the blood pressure of the hypertensive men.

Follow-up research by other investigators has shown that aerobic exercise seems to have its most pervasive effect on dynamic blood pressure. Dynamic blood pressure fluctuates throughout the day due to a person's mood swings and day-to-day pressures. Aerobically fit people will have dramatic blood pressure increases when challenged or upset, just like anybody else. However, their blood pressures will not go as high as expected and their pressures will drop more quickly after the confrontation or emotional upheaval.

Energy-robbing neuromuscular headaches can also be relieved through physical activity. A study conducted by Dr. Herbert deVries of the Gerontology Center at the University of California illustrates this nicely. Working with a group of men 50 years and older, all of whom had a history of migraine headaches, deVries found that after a few weeks of regular physical activity, the headaches disappeared—without medication.

Anger and Anxiety Abatement

Exercise can also play an important role in helping to relieve anger and anxiety. Earlier I shared with you that swatting a handball is good therapy for me. It relieves my frustrations. I know hundreds of other YMCA personnel who have told me the same thing. A vigorous game of racquetball, basketball, or volleyball helps them temper their hostilities and frustrations in a socially acceptable way.

Dr. William P. Morgan, researcher par excellence on emotions and exercise at the University of Wisconsin, noted at a recent conference that after a vigorous workout there is a measurable decrease in anxiety. The level of adrenalin in the blood, the blood pressure, and the heart rate are also reduced. Clinically, many people report improved feelings and less anxiety after a good bout of strenuous exercise.

While it is difficult at the present time to determine how exercise improves the mind and why it reduces anger and anxiety, it probably will be demonstrated in the future that the brain's nerve transmitters are changed in some way that causes people to feel better and more vigorous.

In addition to walking, running, or swatting handballs, there are other ways in which negative emotions caused by stress can be transformed into useful energy. Therapist Laura Archera Huxley has noted that, "We are all links in an infinitely ramifying chain of reactions and events in which people are always passing on irritability and other forms of hostile energy that they have encountered elsewhere." The goal, says Huxley, is to learn to catch this energy as if it were a ball and to use it for a purpose you have chosen. This can be done, she claims, not only through expressive forms of movement such as dance but through any kind of consciously directed, muscular activity. She advocates kicking or squeezing a tether ball, or at moments when one experiences stress but cannot react openly to it, repeatedly contracting for ten seconds, then relaxing muscle groups that one wishes to strengthen or beautify. For example, the abdomen, thighs, or derriere. Such isometric exercises will convert anger or anxiety that's otherwise destined to cause physical or emotional problems into greater fitness and well-being. By retraining ourselves to react to hostile energy with movement of some kind, no matter how subtle, we can become "expert voluntary energy transformers instead of involuntary energy victims."

While I could continue to quote other people and studies on anxiety and anxiousness, I think Dr. Alan Clark of St. Joseph's Infirmary in Atlanta, Georgia, summarizes it best: "It is well known that exercise is the best tranquilizer. I refuse to medicate patients with simple neurotic anxiety until they have given aerobic exercise an adequate trial." Amen!

Depression and Blues

As mentioned earlier, psychologists and psychiatrists are now looking at exercise, specifically running, as an option to help people handle the blues, or mild depression. For some reason, running seems to be a mood elevator. Studies at the University of Virginia among students who claimed to suffer from depression showed that those who worked out vigorously three times a week for ten weeks had an improvement in their scores on tests designed to measure depression. Working out lifted their feelings. The wrestlers, the joggers, the exercisers, and tennis players all noted this mood elevation. But those who played softball did not. It is entirely possible that softball simply isn't vigorous enough to have the effect of reducing depression.

Another study done recently at the University of Wisconsin under the direction of Dr. John Griest compared running with psychotherapy. Although this was only a small-scale, private study, the preliminary data suggests that in some cases running may be as effective as therapy.

In this study people who came to the clinic were assigned to ten weeks of running therapy, ten weeks of psychotherapy, or to unlimited psychotherapy. The running group had to hoof it with their therapist three times a week. Talk of depression was discouraged during the run. If the patient persisted in discussing it, the leader suggested the patient focus on running and breathing instead. At the end of the experiment, the running patients and those in the ten-week psychotherapy group showed the most improvement. Significantly, a year later most of the joggers were still running and were free of depression.

Such changes as raising a person out of depression, reducing anxiety, and transferring stress can make exercising addictive. People find that they need to exercise as much as others need their morning cup of coffee. According to Dr. William Glasser, physician and author of several books, exercise can transform negative addictions into positive ones. Those involved often choose to give up such things as smoking, drinking, overeating, and nonproductive arguing in favor of something more enjoyable and constructive—exercise.

"I have often started out a walk in a state called mad . . ." said Donald Culors Pattie. "Mad in the sense of soreheaded, or mad with tedium or confusion; I have set forth dull, null, and even thoroughly discouraged but I never came back in such a frame of mind, and I have never met a human being that was not better for a walk." This is equally true of other forms of exercise.

Creativity

Allow me to give you a personal illustration. One of the reasons I exercise is because my head calls for it. I may be happy to get the benefits derived from looking better and feeling healthier, but as far as I am concerned they are only side effects. The real reason is mental or emotional. Exercise adds life to my years. It improves my creativity. People ask me, "What keeps you running?" The first 10 minutes of the run, I don't know what keeps me running. Then, I have all kinds of excuses for not running: "I should be back at the office," "My legs hurt," "I don't feel good," "It's cold." The next 20 minutes are for my body. I start to get into rhythm. I realize what is happening to me. I feel my muscles working, my heart beating faster. I like the physical challenge. I'm proud to be exercising. I'm proud that I'm doing something about my physical capabilities. About 30 minutes into my run, my creative juices really start to flow. The LSD starts to take effect. I solve all kinds of administrative, writing, family, and personal problems in a short period of time. Most of my book, program, and article ideas have come on the run. I agree with Dr. George Sheehan who has said, "Never trust an idea that you have sitting down." When my run is finished I am tired physically. But I am full of creative energy. I think I've figured out why this happens. It is time away from the phone, children, and other obligations. Quiet time for myself.

Dr. Thaddeus Kostrubala, the running psychiatrist mentioned earlier, takes it even further. He says that the creative part of my brain has probably taken over. The good doctor notes that as a runner approaches the 30-minute mark, he feels depressed. Some subjects even told him that at the 30-minute mark they feel like crying and occasionally do. Perhaps it is pain, perhaps it is the desire for sympathy. But a short time after the 30-minute mark is reached, some people experience an "opening-up phenomenon." Their breathing becomes easier, their legs feel stronger, and they feel almost euphoric.

Now Kostrubala admits this is a pretty amazing phenomenon. His explanation deals with the left and right sides of the brain. The left side controls the functional aspects of day-to-day living, while the right side controls, among other things, creative functions. The only problem is that to break through to that right side takes some doing. In a sense, we have to escape one level of consciousness to give the brain a clear slate from which to produce new ideas—to create. This level of consciousness is often approached through various forms of repetition. The "OM" of transcendental meditation is one example. Nearly all religions of both East and West utilize a form of repetition to reach a particular level of consciousness, or communion with a higher being.

Kostrubala maintains that the repetitive nature of running, along with whatever repetition you intone mentally with each step, helps you to reach this level of consciousness. He suggests that after 30 or 40 minutes of slow, long-distance, repetitive running, the left side of the brain gets bored and lets the right side of the brain take over. In other words, you have more creative energy. Of course, that phenomenon need not be confined to running. Walking, swimming, bicycling, and cross-country skiing will elicit the same response.

If you feel that this left-right side aspect of the brain is a bunch of mumbo-jumbo, I think you may accept the fact that exercise improves your creative processes for the following reasons.

A lot of times our busy schedules prevent us from periods of reflection necessary to the creative process. We get all wrapped up in our daily routine and do things out of habit. We know we should spend more time alone thinking, perhaps meditating, but we are filled with so much nervous energy that we can't sit still. Here's where exercise helps. The calm solitude of exercising alone outdoors gives you a chance to work things out in your mind. New ideas, to help you approach old problems, are more likely to pop into your head while you are running, cycling, or walking, than if you spent the same time watching TV or worrying about that problem.

Confidence

Good fitness builds confidence as well. Dr. Thomas K. Cureton, the granddaddy of fitness in the U.S.A., says that this is one of the greatest benefits of exercise. His exhaustive work at the University of Illinois over four decades convinced him that most middle-age men lose confidence in their physical ability as they get older. They become unfit, have sagging waistlines, flabby muscles, gain weight, and are breathless under exertion. Many are afraid that increased physical activity might injure them or precipitate a heart attack. They literally lose their physical ego. Since men are taught early in life that manliness and physical vigor go hand in hand, their self-confidence slips. And when this slips, their mental and emotional areas are affected as well.

Cureton maintains that through exercise men will lose their timidity. As their narrow waistline returns, weight drops, muscles firm up, and stamina improves, they become physical beings once more. Exercise helps them to reestablish their self-confidence.

I must admit, however, that these feelings are sometimes dangerous. People have reported to me that they are deluded with feelings of power when they become fit. They actually feel that they can meet a truck head-on and win the battle. It is conceivable that this change may be due to hyperventilation —rapid breathing that over-oxygenates the blood. But for the most part it's probably due to Cureton's contention that they become physical beings once more. They literally return to their days of their youth and enjoy being a physical person.

How to Do It

I hope by now you are excited enough about the possibility of gaining more energy through aerobic exercise to give it a try. But don't just lace on a pair of sneakers and head for the hills. Unfortunately, too many people get all hyped up about exercise, overdo it, then suffer minor problems like blisters and aching muscles. Such negative experiences usually turn them off. Instead, you need to approach your exercise program more realistically. To begin with, establish how much, how hard, and how often you should exercise.

How Much

Don't get hung up on distance. A mistake many people make when they begin a walking or jogging program is to measure their distance. Miles don't mean a thing to your body. Minutes do. If you have been inactive for at least a year, I suggest setting a goal of 20 to 30 minutes of aerobic activity. If it's longer than that, you will probably push too hard and may suffer some minor aches and pains. As you become more proficient and your fitness level increases, you can increase that time up to an hour a day if you choose. However, as far as increased energy and general fitness is concerned, 30 to 40 minutes of aerobic exercise each session is an adequate amount.

How Hard

You have an amazing mechanism for determining how hard to exercise: your pulse. The first thing you should learn in beginning a program of aerobic exercise is to listen to your body. And the first place to listen is your wrist. Use the second, third, and fourth fingers of one hand to feel for the pulse along the thumb-side of your other wrist. Take your pulse rate for ten seconds. This count should then be multiplied by six to find out how many times your heart beats per minute.

Go ahead and try to take your pulse now. You'll probably find it's between 60 and 80 beats per minute. It's relatively easy to take your pulse while sitting, but when you're outside swimming, bicycling, or running, you'll have to stop for a few seconds, check your pulse, and then resume your activity.

How does this tell you how hard you should exercise? Your ideal exercise level is determined by your target heart rate. Your target heart rate is approximately 70 to 85 percent of your maximum heart rate (see below). To make sure you are exercising hard enough, check your pulse occasionally to see if your heart rate falls within the target zone. The maximum heart rate of a young child is around 220 beats per minute, and since physiologists tell us that our maximum heart rate drops about one beat a year, you can subtract your age from the maximum number of 220 beats per minute. So if you are 40 years of age, your maximum heart rate would be 180. To find your target heart rate, simply figure 70 to 85 percent of that number. This is how the target heart rate chart below was determined.

Age	Target Heart Rate (Beats per Minute)
10–19	145 to 180
20–29	140 to 170

30–39	130 to 160
40–49	125 to 150
50–59	115 to 140
60–69	105 to 130

In addition to monitoring your pulse rate, you can determine whether you are exercising too hard by listening to other parts of your body. If your breathing is extremely labored or if you feel a tightness or pain in your chest or shoulder, then you should slow down. A good guide is to determine whether you are able to hold a conversation while exercising. If you are breathing so hard that you can't talk, then you are working too hard. The secret of success is to listen carefully to your body.

By listening to your body you can forget the stopwatch. One of the most destructive forces in a good maximum personal energy exercise program is trying to beat the clock. You figure if two miles in 17 minutes is good, then two miles in 15 minutes is even better. That kind of thinking will drain your energy, not build it. Think in terms of exercising for a period of time when you feel good. Constantly pushing yourself to be number one can drain you physically and frustrate you unless you have inherited O. J. Simpson's genes.

Remember, you are exercising for maximum personal energy, not for sport. When you run, bike, swim, or walk against the clock as part of trying to excel in competition, you have moved from fitness to sport. Your goal in building energy is to go long and slow.

How Often

How often is really quite simple to decide. As a rule, three days per week is the minimum. You simply must commit yourself to that minimum if you are interested in increasing your energy level. While some people try to exercise every day of the week, usually a day or two of rest is advisable, especially if you have been inactive for some time. So your prescription for higher energy through aerobic exercise includes 20 to 40 minutes of target heart rate exercise three to six days a week.

Also, do your exercising in a relaxed manner. Don't focus constantly on the clock. Don't be highly competitive. Your world is probably competitive enough. Making your sport or physical activity competitive can turn it into an energy-robber. Be relaxed in your approach to fitness. Enjoy!

CHAPTER 10
Stretch for Energy

It feels good to stretch. It's relaxing. It's a symbol of contentment. On Saturday morning when you roll out of bed late and aren't in a particular rush to be somewhere by a certain time, a lazy yawn escapes you, accompanied by a slow groan and a nice, refreshing stretch. Without even thinking, you reach for the ceiling, bend those elbows, flex those shoulders and rotate the head to work that kink out of your neck. Then you rub it gently and mumble, "Humm, musta slept funny."

What do you do after a filling, delicious meal? You try to control the belch, but the deep breath, the contented sigh, and the involuntary chest stretching are perfectly acceptable. Your host knows that you are pleased, and somehow you really feel good.

If you were not allowed to stretch at all for a week, you'd begin to feel like a walking time bomb. Tension would mount, muscles would become impossibly stiff, and your range of motion would be severely restricted. You would be seriously affected emotionally and psychologically, as well as physically. The stretch reflex allows you to relax.

Human beings love to stretch, they can't cope with life for long without stretching, and fortunately, stretching is very good for them. A little stretching is essential, and a lot of stretching, if done properly, can do no harm. In fact, it can result in greater physical efficiency, coordination, agility, balance and quickness, a vastly improved range of motion, and most importantly, a release of muscle tension. As a consequence, it is the best insurance you can have against injury. The fringe benefit is that *proper* stretching is one of the best relaxation techniques there is.

115

Athletes are dedicated stretchers, primarily because they know it's the best way to avoid winding up being carried off the field on a stretcher. Most torn ligaments, pulled muscles, and other bodily injuries due to vigorous movement could be prevented by a proper warm-up that includes careful stretching of the various muscle groups.

Dr. George A. Sheehan, M.D., reports: "Although most athletes, fans, and physicians still view such tragedies (muscle pulls, tears, and strains) as acts of God, there is a growing awareness that these injuries are not accidental, that they can even be predicted and prevented."

Many pro football teams are convinced this is true and now employ "flex" coaches who direct players in stretching exercises.

So stretch for energy, because there's nothing like an injury (unless it's a disease) to make you suddenly feel energy-deficient. Just a hangnail can make you feel bad all over. You can imagine what Achilles tendonitis will do for your energy level.

You're probably not an athlete though, and aren't likely to get seriously damaged as they are. However, you have just read a chapter on aerobic exercise and its value. So you want to get started. But you're wondering if stretching is to be part of that program.

The answer is absolutely yes! I recommend ten minutes of stretching as part of the warm-up before any aerobic activity, to reduce the possibility of injury. Following the workout, do ten minutes of stretching as part of your cool-down to prevent stiff, sore muscles, and to help you relax. In fact, though the injury prevention qualities of proper stretching cannot be overemphasized, it's the contribution stretching makes to relaxation that most fascinates me. You can stretch to relax, and the result will be less tension, less fatigue, less exhaustion. In fact, many people who practice stretching, yoga, or similar kinds of activities report that afterwards they are more vigorous and alert. In other words, they have more energy.

To achieve relaxation requires that you take time on a regular basis to reduce your physical tension. Many people are unaware of how badly they need to relax. They have lived the fast-paced, high-strung life for so long that they think their tension is normal. Sure, they have vague feelings of discomfort, have trouble getting rest, are easily irritated, and develop periodic aches, pains, and headaches. Doesn't everyone? Everyone does once in a while, but when it gets chronic, it's probably due to tension.

Some of the more obvious strategies for coping with stress are to swear a lot, blame your feelings on others, or throw things. The results of these strategies are seldom beneficial, however, for they only lead to more tension, and guilt feelings. A better approach is to take time for isolation and meditation, talk your tensions through with a friend, or find a funny distraction or bit of entertainment at which to laugh. Laughing is very relaxing.

These are all psychological aids to relaxing, and all very good. A frequently overlooked way of relaxing, unwinding, and building of energy, though, is through stretching. Yoga enthusiasts have expounded this aspect of their activity for years, but only recently have scientists come to realize its true benefits.

The Benefits of Stretching

The main jobs your muscles have to do are to tighten or contract. The contraction allows limbs to move so you can run, walk, sit, stand, eat, write, type, and drive. Tension is necessary for every move you make. It is normal and necessary. Of course, muscles are not to be tense or contracted all the time. When sitting, the muscles of your upper legs are generally relaxed, as are your abdominal muscles. But your lower back and lower leg muscles are contracted to help you sit properly. When lying down, however, your thigh muscles are contracted and your back muscles are relaxed. This beautiful interplay of muscles relaxing, contracting, and partially contracting or relaxing allows you to function efficiently and smoothly with minimum fatigue.

Since your muscles make up a major portion of your body weight (over 60 percent), and respond quickly to the fight or flight phenomenon of your sympathetic nervous system and endocrine system, the muscles are usually the first sign of tension. Before you have a headache, stomach pain, or whipped feeling, your muscles warn you with an eye twitch, a neck or back pain, or muscle fatigue.

Problems result when muscles tense up and there is no need for the tension. There's no reason for your back muscles to be tight when you're lying down. However, many people do remain tense even in prone positions, which ought to explain why low back pain is one of the major complaints doctors hear about these days. A majority of back problems are the result of weak or inflexible muscles; muscles that stay tight even though they ought to be relaxing.

To find out if your muscles are too tense, pay attention to these warning signs:

1. Do you have eye twitches?
2. Do you have neck or low back pain?
3. Do you have restless legs (you feel as though you must get up and walk about frequently)?

4. Do you seem to clench your fists repeatedly? Or do you hold the phone or steering wheel of your car very tightly?
5. Do your muscles seem to tire more easily when performing a physical task—such as typing and writing?
6. Do you seem to lack flexibility at different joints of your body? When you try to touch your toes do your back and leg muscles rebel?
7. Upon awakening, does it seem as though your jaw is tired as a result of gritting or clenching your teeth?
8. Do you find that you have been very rigid in your sleeping?
9. Does your spouse tell you that you twitch or jump a great deal?

All of these are symptoms of muscle tension. And if they occur infrequently, it's not too much of a problem. But if they appear repetitively during a week, then you know that you're probably experiencing too much muscle tension.

Once you've discovered that you have muscle tension and fatigue, it's time to use stretching for relaxation, reducing fatigue, and hence, building energy.

The Two Types of Stretching

Exercise physiologists tell us there are two basic stretching methods: ballistic and static. Ballistic stretching involves bouncing and bobbing to see how close you can come to touching your toes. Static stretching is the slow, easy approach where you gradually reach down to the point where you feel a tug on your muscles. At that point you hold. Then you concentrate on the tight muscle groups, trying to get these muscles to relax. The muscles usually relax and then you can slip down a little bit further to another point of tug or slight discomfort. This position is then to be held for approximately ten seconds. Over the weeks the point of tug or discomfort should be reduced, permitting you to go a little bit further. The result is an improvement of flexibility, the by-product of relaxed muscles.

Opinions differ on which is best—ballistic or static stretching. If your physical education teacher in high school was an ex-marine from World War II or the Korean War, then you did ballistic stretching in the old "hup . . . two . . . three . . . four" routine. More recently, static stretching has been employed with good success among professional athletic teams. In fact, it has become so pervasive among athletic teams that many have entirely rejected the old ballistic routines.

To discover which approach is best, Dr. Herbert deVries of the University of Southern California undertook an investigation. His research concluded that static stretching is just as effective as the old-fashioned ballistic method, but there are three distinct advantages to static stretching:

1. There's less danger of exceeding the extensibility limits of the tissues involved (less chance of injury and pain).
2. Static stretching requires less energy.
3. Ballistic stretching is likely to cause muscular soreness, but static stretching will not. In fact, static stretching generally relieves sore muscles.

Interestingly, deVries also discovered that the improvements brought about by static stretching persisted for a longer period of time—eight weeks and more—after the stretching program was discontinued. Significantly, stretching can improve the flexibility and relaxation ability in the old as well as in the young.

If you are familiar with exercise, you'll probably recognize that static stretching is similar to the classic yoga poses, postures, and concepts. And it is the static stretch that I recommend for a warm-up prior to aerobic exercise and cool-down after exercise. I also recommend static stretching as a relaxation technique.

Back in the 1960s, in their quest for a more fulfilled life, reduced tension, and a desire for greater energy reserves, many Americans turned to yoga. There are many varieties of yoga, but the most popular type is Hatha Yoga. In Hatha (physical) Yoga, a series of postures (asanas) consisting of stretching, head and shoulder stands, balancing, standing, and sitting postures is employed. A yoga workout typically combines groups of these postures (to stretch most major muscle groups), the movements of getting into and out of them, relaxation, and simple breathing exercises. A great deal of emphasis is placed on static stretching. Many yogis are in the habit of placing their bodies in what you might consider extremely uncomfortable positions for as long as 20 to 30 minutes a day. While there is nothing wrong with that, it is not necessary for you to hold stretch positions that long for either your warm-ups to aerobic exercise or for relaxation. Ten seconds to one minute for each stretch exercise is enough.

What does stretching have to do with your energy? According to Richard Hittleman, the most prolific U.S. writer on the subject, "The results of the practice of Hatha Yoga are equated with what are supposed to be the characteristics of youth." He adds that "people who practice yoga will have improved: flexibility; grace; serenity; relaxation; sleep; vitality; endurance; circulation;

strength of vital organs and glands; firmness and strength of muscles; taut, smooth skin; weight; recovery; alertness; and clarity of mind."

That's quite a list of benefits, and it stretches the facts. Research does not support all of these avid contentions. Although I will be discussing the energy-giving benefits of Hatha Yoga in particular, realize that the benefits of static stretching are similar, whether derived from yoga or any other static stretching program. Remember, however, that yogis spend long hours in static stretch positions in their quest to obtain these benefits. I feel similar benefits may be derived by holding the static stretch position for no more than a minute or so. Devote the time you save to an activity that burns calories and has a training effect on your heart and lungs. Ultimately this will build greater energy.

Researchers state that yoga postures will do the following: decrease oxygen consumption, respiration, resting heart rate, blood pressure, and muscle tension. All the while it also increases the intensity of the brain's alpha waves.

The decrease in oxygen consumption is fascinating. Oxygen consumption refers to your metabolic rate. Each cell uses the energy (calories) in the food by slowly burning these nutrients. This requires oxygen. So the bloodstream delivers oxygen to the cells. The sum of all your cells using oxygen is called your total oxygen consumption, or the metabolism of your body. Research shows that yoga-type activities decrease a person's metabolic rate. Decreased metabolic rate is what physiologists would call a restful state. Like sleep, yoga permits the body to be taxed less—a chance for you to "recharge your batteries."

People who live on hype all the time, who are high strung, do 15 things at once, struggle with their station in life, and live on what seems like perpetual energy soon find that their bodies become tense. The increased respiration rate, heart rate, blood pressure, and muscle tension that accompany their hyperactivity increase oxygen consumption. Their metabolism may soar very high for an extended period of time, but eventually it needs a recharge. Relaxation exercises such as stretching provide that avenue through decreasing the symptoms of hyperactivity.

Alpha waves, however, are another story. Alpha waves are your slow brain waves. They increase in intensity when you do yoga. Scientists are still at a loss on how to explain the exact role of the alpha waves, but they do know that alpha waves are more abundant in people who feel relaxed. Yoga increases those waves.

Interestingly, yoga practitioners also demonstrate lower activity of the sympathetic nervous system. In Chapter 5 I related how the sympathetic nervous system, while it does give you a lift with respect to energy, can eventually let you down if overtaxed.

To derive the most benefit from stretching, be sure to do it correctly. Hittleman notes, and other yogis agree, that you are to do each stretch slowly and without straining. Don't worry if you cannot achieve the extreme positions of the super-flexible individual. Stretch only as far as is comfortable. While you are holding that position, relax. When you feel tension in a particular muscle, concentrate on relaxing it. Remarkably, this advice on stretching in yoga is parallel to the results suggested by deVries' research: the stretch is to be slow, sustained, and not ballistic.

Research, logic, and experience indicate that yoga exercises are very effective in improving flexibility. Caution must be exercised, however, not to get into extreme positions without proper conditioning. Dr. Allan Ryan, in his critique on yoga, wrote, "Unsupervised attempts . . . to assume some of the more difficult postures might result in some harm to the untrained individual." The same is true of other stretches. Extreme postures are not necessary for the average person. However, don't avoid stretching entirely either. Anyone on an aerobic program of running, walking, or cycling should definitely use selected static stretch exercises for flexibility development.

The nice things about static stretching are that no special exercise devices are needed, you can work at your own rate, and you can choose the exercises that meet your special needs. Paul Uram, the flex coach for the Pittsburgh Steelers, has made many suggestions and observations about proper stretching, some of which follow.

1. Do not force your muscles to stretch more than they are ready for, and don't progress too rapidly.
2. When stretching one set of muscles, also stretch the opposite set. That is, when you stretch the hamstring muscles, also stretch the quadricep muscles.
3. The functioning of one muscle group is almost always related to the functioning of another group, so that stretches to help the back may also benefit both leg and shoulder muscles.
4. Keep warm while stretching. This enhances all of the benefits of static stretches.
5. Learn to recognize the tension, discomfort, and sometimes actual pain that accompany stretching, and use it to your advantage. It's a form of feedback that can help you recognize how far you can safely stretch. While performing a given stretch, go far enough to derive some benefit but not so far that you damage yourself. Each time you do a given stretch you can lean on the muscles a bit more to gradually improve your

flexibility. By paying close attention to the various sorts of discomfort that you feel, you will learn to recognize the tensions that are normal and safe. Other tensions can be relaxed or exercised away. Severe tensions are painful and require rest or special treatment. These can be avoided by means of careful stretching.

6. Relax while stretching. Don't hold your breath. Breathe normally. Rather than fighting the exercise, relax your way through it.

7. Hold stretches for short periods of time at first and then progress to longer holds.

8. DO NOT BOUNCE. Bouncing does not allow the muscle time to benefit from the stretch, and it is dangerous and may cause injury. Also, bouncing actually causes the muscle to contract rather than to adapt to the stretched length, due to what is called the stretch reflex. Since most sports and aerobic exercises are ballistic in nature, a type of stretching that counteracts that activity is recommended. Consequently, static stretching is recommended. Ballistic stretching should be avoided.

9. If you do not have the flexibility and poise of a gymnast, don't let that stop you from beginning a stretch program. It makes no difference how flexible you are. Don't compare yourself with others. Just stretch *your* muscles, and learn to like that stretching feeling. Hold each stretch in a position that is fairly comfortable but that still exerts some tension. Hold that position until you feel yourself relax. Never strain. There is no way your body can relax if you are straining.

As far as I'm concerned, aerobic exercise and static stretching make the perfect marriage for building energy. One builds energy by increasing the oxygen-carrying capacity of your body, building better muscle tone, developing a better cardiovascular system that functions more efficiently, reducing your body fat, helping reduce the blues, and giving an outlet for removing your anger and anxiety. Static stretching, on the other hand, complements aerobic exercise and gives you an opportunity to maintain your flexibility so that you can do plenty of aerobic exercise for true relaxation. It winds you down from the hype of a busy life.

Many aerobic exercisers forget the importance of stretching. They go into the activity full bore. In my fitness classes around the United States and in my consultations at YMCAs I see many men who come rushing in from their office at 12 noon, tie ajar. They quickly undress, get into their gym shorts, and bound up to the gymnasium to start doing their laps. As soon as the aerobic exercise is finished, they rush back to the locker room, down a few glasses of juice or a cup of yogurt, and dash off to the office. While they may be building aerobic fitness, they have done nothing to help prevent injury. On top of it they have not really relaxed. They have been under the gun the whole time. While they're building one type of aerobic energy, I'm afraid they're just adding more hype to their life. They must learn to approach the activity in a more relaxed manner. Stretching provides that opportunity.

Yogis are many times at fault as well. They forget about aerobic exercise. They think stretching will do it all. Stretching will provide relaxation. But they forget that a more healthful cardiovascular system will help to build energy by increasing their body's ability to pick up and transport oxygen. Of course, many yogis point with pride to cats. They note that cats stretch all the time and yet are in fantastic shape. But they forget to point out that the cat is also an aerobic animal. It runs, leaps, hops, climbs, jumps, and has an unbelievable aerobic capacity. A cat is probably the perfect animal. It stretches, runs, and stretches. As a result, it is fit and has a tremendous amount of stamina.

So put the two together. Stretch and become fit aerobically.

Stretching Techniques

Below are a series of stretches that I recommend. They are a blend of traditional movements and yoga postures, poses, and breathing. These stretches are followed by our three phase program for improving your energy via exercise.

Moderate Stretching Exercises

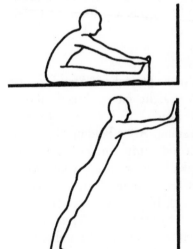

Sitting Toe Touches—Sit with legs extended in front of you, feet together, and legs flat on the floor. Reach for toes with hands, bringing forehead as close to knees as possible.

Calf Tendon Stretcher—Stand 2 to 3 feet from the wall. Lean forward, body straight. Place palms against the wall at eye level. Step backward. Continue to support your weight with hands. Remain flat-footed until you feel calf muscles stretching.

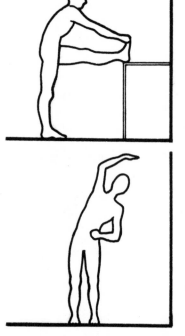

Standing Leg Stretcher—Find a chair or table 2½ to 3 feet in height. Place left foot on the chair or table. Keep this leg straight and parallel to the floor. Your right leg should be planted firmly on the floor. From this position, slowly extend your fingertips toward your outstretched leg on the chair. Hold and return. Eventually you should get forehead to knee. Repeat with your other leg.

Side-to-Side Stretch—Stand with feet shoulder-width apart, left hand at your side, right hand extended over your head. Slowly bend at the waist toward your left. Reach down your leg with your left hand. Try to get your upper body parallel to the floor. Hold for eight to ten seconds, then repeat in the other direction.

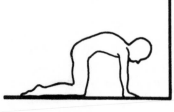

Cat Stretch—Get on your hands and knees and take a few relaxing breaths. Then, curl your chin to your chest, while arching your back. Hold that position for eight to ten seconds, then relax.

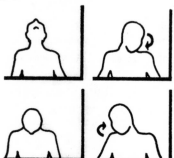

Simple Neck Stretches—Stand or sit with your back straight, facing directly ahead. Slowly tilt your head up as if to look at something on the ceiling. After holding that position for ten seconds, turn and look over your left shoulder without twisting your upper body. Hold for ten seconds, then turn to the right. Again, hold, then look down, trying to touch your chin to your chest. This exercise can be practiced several times throughout the day and is a great way to reduce neck muscle tension that can lead to headaches.

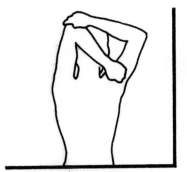

Shoulder Stretch—With your arms over your head, hold the elbow of one arm with the hand of the other arm. Slowly pull the elbow behind your head. Do not force. Hold. Repeat on the other side.

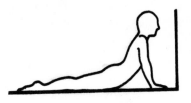

Abdomen Stretch—Lie face down on the floor, hands flat against the floor beside your chest in a push-up position. Relax. Then slowly push your upper body off the floor, looking up toward the ceiling. Continue pushing until you feel slight pressure in your abdomen. Hold. Lower your body slowly to the floor.

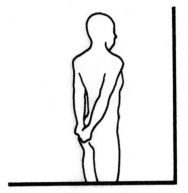

Bend and Stretch—While standing, clasp hands behind your waist. As you slowly bend forward at the waist, lift your arms, keeping the elbows straight. When you begin to feel slight pressure, stop and hold. Return to starting position.

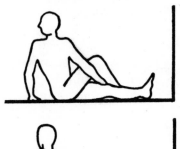

Simple Body Twist—Sit with your left leg extended, your right leg crossed over so that right foot is on the outside of the left knee. Place left hand against the outside of the left knee, right hand on the floor beside the right hip. Now turn your upper body to the right, trying to look over your right shoulder. Hold, then repeat on the other side.

Yoga Stretches

A good way to begin a yoga stretching session is with the classic "Greeting the Sun" series of poses. This exercise will stretch the spine and tendons, help you to breathe regularly, get rid of unwanted fat, and provide steady, moderate exercise for your heart.

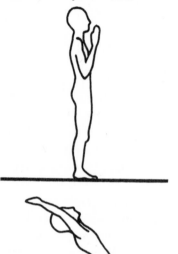

1. Stand erect with your feet together. Put your palms together in front of your chest. Relax your body as you prepare to learn the 12 poses. Eventually, you will do them almost automatically, as one long, smooth, flowing movement. Breathe naturally as you rest your mind and body.

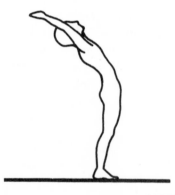

2. Raise your arms with palms facing each other, stretching them back over your head, slightly apart, and arch your body slightly backwards. Imagine yourself stretching in the sun's rays and receiving its warmth and energy. Breathe in slowly as you raise your arms.

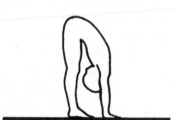

3. Bend forward, touching your hands flat to the floor (if you can without bouncing) in front of your feet, keeping your legs straight. Let your head hang down and be relaxed. Breathe out as you bend forward, emptying your lungs as you pull your stomach up.

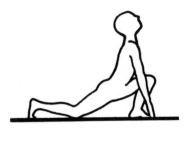

4. Move your right leg back, letting your right knee touch the floor, while your hands and left foot remain in the same position as the previous pose and your left knee bends forward. Rest your head on the back of your neck, stretching the whole front of your body slightly. Breathe in as you move your leg back.

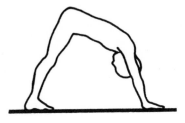

5. Place your left leg beside your right leg, push your buttocks up, pull your head down between your shoulders. Your arms, torso, and legs form a triangle with the floor. Attempt to keep your heels on the floor. Breathe out as you bring your left leg alongside your right leg.

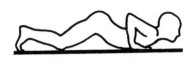

6. Lower your body to the floor, allowing your chin, chest, knees, feet, and hands to contact the floor. Keep your buttocks, thighs, and abdomen off the floor. Breathe out before you lower your body and then, as you lower your body hold your breath, and remain in this pose.

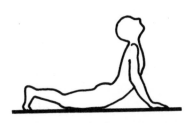

7. Bend your upper torso and head backwards, until your arms are straight. Breathe in deeply as you bend backwards.

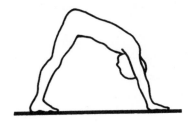

8. Push your buttocks up again until you form a triangle with the floor. Breathe out as you form a triangle.

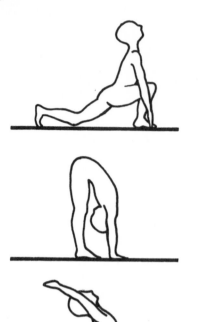

9. Move your right leg forward, bending it at the knee until your right foot rests on the floor between your hands, resting your head back on your neck and looking up toward the center of your brow. Breathe in as you move your right leg.

10. Bring your left foot forward and straighten your legs without taking your hands off the floor. Bend forward, pushing your head between your shoulders. Breathe out as you bend forward.

11. Stretch your arms back over your head as you raise your torso and slightly arch your back (same as Pose 2). Breathe in deeply as you stretch backwards.

12. Bring your hands down to your chest and stand erect and relaxed. Breathe naturally.

At first, this series will take some practice until you have memorized the sequence. Once you have it memorized, move through it a bit more rapidly so that your breathing becomes more forceful. Always go through it at least twice, alternating legs when you put one foot forward. To make it more aerobic in nature, go through it several times each session.

Other Yoga Stretches

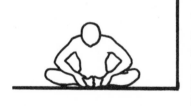

Knee and Thigh Stretch—Sit on the floor with your knees bent, heels pulled up toward your buttocks. Place the soles of your feet together and clasp your hands firmly around your feet. Pull up on your feet with your hands, trying to drop your thighs and knees as far downward as possible. Hold, breathing deeply.

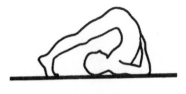

Plough—Lie flat on your back with your arms at your sides. Turn your palms downward so that they press against the floor. Bring your legs together and slowly raise them until they extend back over your head, parallel to the floor. Continue to push down on the floor with your hands. When you come out of this position, make sure you bend your knees and keep them close to your head as you roll back to the beginning position.

Rishi's Posture—Stand with feet shoulder-width apart. Stretch both arms directly in front of you, palms facing the floor, parallel to the ground. Slowly twist your upper body to the right, arms pointing in the direction you turn. When you have reached as far as you can, hold for ten seconds. Return to the starting position, breathe deeply, then twist to the left.

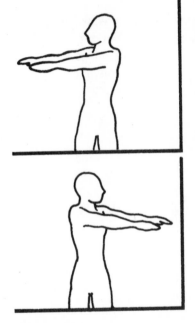

The Yogic "Complete Breath" Breathing Technique

1. Sit in a cross-legged posture. Relax and breathe normally. Begin by using your abdominal muscles to push your abdomen out as far as possible while inhaling as deeply as possible.
2. Practice pulling in with the abdomen and pushing out the air, first in the lower chest, then in the upper chest areas. Finally, raise your shoulders, keeping your hands on your knees.
3. Slowly lower your shoulders and relax your chest and abdomen.
4. Practice to make Step 1 flow easily into Step 2.

5. Now, practice the breathing again. Exhale through your nose until you completely empty your lungs. Then, slowly inhale so that it takes 15 seconds to fill your lungs.
6. Retain the air in your lungs for 10 seconds.
7. Exhale through your nose, taking 15 seconds to allow the air to slowly escape.
8. Repeat Steps 5, 6, and 7 until the 15-10-15 second counting is mastered.
9. Make sure you coordinate the breathing with the movements of your abdomen.

Whether you decide to try some of the yoga stretches, or to rely on the more traditional stretches described earlier, you will enhance your energy level by including some planned stretching in your daily routine. Not only will it help you to relax, it will prepare your body for the physical demands it must face. Combined with regular aerobic activity, stretching will give you an energy edge against fatigue.

A Three Phase Plan for Enjoying Fitness

Take the following tests to see how fit you are:

Cooper's Three-Mile Walking Test (No Running)

Time (Minutes)

Fitness Category	Age (Years)					
	13–19	20–29	30–39	40–49	50–59	60+
I. Very Poor						
(Men)	>45:00*	>46:00	>49:00	>52:00	>55:00	>60:00
(Women)	>47:00	>48:00	>51:00	>54:00	>57:00	>63:00
II. Poor						
(Men)	41:01–45:00	42:01–46:00	44:31–49:00	47:01–52:00	50:01–55:00	54:01–60:00
(Women)	43:01–47:00	44:01–48:00	46:31–51:00	49:01–54:00	52:01–57:00	57:01–63:00
III. Fair						
(Men)	37:31–41:00	38:31–42:00	40:01–44:30	42:01–47:00	45:01–50:00	48:01–54:00
(Women)	39:31–43:00	40:31–44:00	42:01–46:30	44:01–49:00	47:01–52:00	51:01–57:00
IV. Good						
(Men)	33:00–37:30	34:00–38:30	35:00–40:00	36:30–42:00	39:00–45:00	41:00–48:00
(Women)	35:00–39:30	36:00–40:30	37:30–42:00	39:00–44:00	42:00–47:00	45:00–51:00
V. Excellent						
(Men)	<33:00	<34:00	<35:00	<36:30	<39:00	<41:00
(Women)	<35:00	<36:00	<37:30	<39:00	<42:00	<45:00

SOURCE: Kenneth H. Cooper, *The Aerobics Way* (New York: M. Evans and Co., 1977).
NOTE: *The Walking Test,* covering three miles in the fastest time possible *without running,* can be done on a track over any accurately measured distance. As with running, take the test after you have been training for at least six weeks, when you feel rested, and dress to be comfortable.
* < means "less than"; > means "more than."

Standard Flexibility Test (Sit and Reach Test)

Materials: yardstick and adhesive tape.

Procedure: 1. Warm up with some stretching before the test.
2. Sit on the floor with the legs extended and the heels about 5 inches apart.
3. With a strip of adhesive tape, mark where the heels touch the floor. The heels should touch the near edge of the tape.
4. Place the yardstick on the floor between and parallel to the legs so that the 15-inch mark touches the near edge of the taped heel line.
5. Slowly reach with both hands as far forward as possible. Touch the fingertips to the yardstick and hold this position momentarily. The yardstick shows the distance reached. *Do not attempt to add length by jerking forward.*

Plan for Enjoying Fitness—Continued

6. Try the test three times, recording the distance in inches each time: _____, _____, _____. Circle your best score.
7. Check your scores with the norms provided.

Rating	Men (Inches)	Women (Inches)
Excellent	22–23	24–27
Good	20–21	21–23
Average	14–18	16–20
Fair	12–13	13–16
Poor	10–11	0–12

SOURCE: C.R. Myers, *The Official YMCA Physical Fitness Handbook* (New York: Popular Library, 1975), pp. 103–104.

The point on the plan at which you begin depends upon how you scored on the Three-Mile Walking Test. If you scored Very Poor or Poor, begin at Phase One. If you scored Fair or Good, begin at Phase Two. If you scored Excellent, begin at Phase Three unless it seems too taxing. In that event, begin about halfway through Phase Two.

Phase One

Flexibility—Spend five minutes a day doing five of the stretching exercises described in Chapter 10.

Aerobic Fitness—Spend at least one week on each of these levels and try to do the activity at least three times each week. If you move up to the next level after a week and it seems too difficult, drop back to the previous level for another week. When you walk, walk at a comfortable yet steady pace. Since you are not in peak physical condition, the most important lesson you can learn is PATIENCE. Moving too rapidly through the levels may result in discomfort or injury.

Number of Minutes to Walk Per Day
10–20
20–25
25–30
30–35
35–40
40–45

Spend a *minimum* of one week at each of these levels.

Plan for Enjoying Fitness—Continued
Phase Two

Flexibility—Spend five minutes twice a day on seven of the stretching exercises described in Chapter 10.

Aerobic Fitness—Spend at least two weeks on each of these levels and try to work out at least four times each week. To determine your target heart rate, subtract your age from 220 (to obtain your maximum rate), then compute 75 percent of that number. Or consult Cooper's Three-Mile Walking test at the beginning of the plan. Walking may be used as a target heart rate activity if you move at a brisk enough pace. Then finish your workout by walking at a more relaxed pace.

Number of Minutes at Target Heart Rate Activity	Number of Minutes to Walk
10	35
12	30
14	25
16	20
18	15
20	10

Spend a *minimum* of two weeks at each level.

Phase Three

Flexibility—Spend ten minutes, twice a day incorporating all the stretching exercises described in Chapter 10, including the yoga stretches. If you are using running as your target heart rate activity, stretching becomes even more important since running causes the muscles along the back of the leg to shorten. Runners may need to stretch more than the suggested amount of time.

Aerobic Fitness—Your entire workout should consist of target heart rate activity and you should aim for a minimum of four days a week. Begin your workout with five minutes of warm-up activity (walking, running in place, or very slow jogging) and end it with a five minute cool-down (walking, stretching). Spend four weeks at each level.

Number of minutes of target heart rate activity
20–25
25–30
30–35

Plan for Enjoying Fitness—Continued

35–40
40–45
45–50
50–55
55–60

Spend a *minimum* of four weeks at each level.

EATING
FOR ENERGY

CHAPTER 11
The Energy Givers

I can't just give you a simple formula for eating. For too long, nutritionists have simply said, "Don't eat this," or "Eat this and that." At other times they have tried to be too simplistic—the four basic food groups are a perfect example. How do you classify such fabricated foods as lasagna, cocktail cheese puffs, imitation cream, vegetable-protein bacon chips, or egg substitutes?

Regarding sugar, there are contradictory opinions. Some say sugar is good for you. It gives you energy. The word from others is, "Avoid sugar completely." The truth lies somewhere between these extremes.

The purpose of this chapter is to explain why there may be good and bad forms of sugar when it comes to energy levels, as well as why certain forms of sugar or starch may enhance your energy levels. To explain this, I need to take you inside your body's complex biochemical system and show you what happens when, for example, you eat a candy bar. If you're a speed reader this chapter may slow you down a trifle, but when you're done you'll have a good handle on how proper eating can contribute a lot toward maximum energy.

Food is energy—if you eat the right kind. Unfortunately, most people don't understand how or what foods provide you with energy. To add to the problem, nutritionists have a different concept of nutrition than you and I do. To them food energy is the number of units of energy in a particular food. Units of energy are called kilocalories, hereafter called calories. A calorie is the amount of heat required to raise the temperature of one kilogram of water one degree centigrade—clear as mud. A more effective definition is given by Fergus M. Clydesdale, professor of Food Service and Nutrition at the University of Massachusetts. He says a calorie is "a unit of energy going into the body and supplying it with a certain amount of power, just as gas powers a car."

Why is this power needed by cells? Cells act as chemical processing plants. Cells take the various chemicals and foods and build them into certain substances. Then they tear these substances back down. This type of activity requires energy or fuel, just as your car needs fuel for it to function. But there is a hitch. A calorie itself is not actually fuel or food for the body. Instead, it is an abstract measurement, like an inch or a pound.

How do you know the number of calories in a particular food? You burn them and then measure the amount of heat given off. The burning is done in what scientists call a bomb calorimeter. Here you set fire to the food and simply burn it. The heat produced is then converted into calories. Simple enough. To do every food in this way, however, would be laborious. So scientists did research that showed that one gram (about $\frac{1}{28}$ of an ounce) of pure carbohydrate contains four calories. One gram of protein contains four calories. One gram of fat contains nine calories.

Since all foods are comprised of some combination of carbohydrates, fats, and proteins, a nutritionist or physiologist can calculate the number of calories in a particular food by determining the percentage of weight of the food that is carbohydrate, fat, and protein. So the next time you read a label of an eight-ounce fruit yogurt container that says there are 260 calories, you know that it was determined by a thorough analysis of the carbohydrate, fat, and protein content of the yogurt.

Contrary to what some people think, it doesn't matter to your body where these calories come from. Your body reads a calorie as a calorie as a calorie. It either uses these calories immediately in the cell for cell activity, or stores it on the body in the form of glycogen, a pretty name for starch. Consequently, your body is a virtual storehouse of energy, just waiting to be tapped.

The quality and amounts of food that you eat have a direct bearing on your energy. Carbohydrates, fats, and proteins, assisted by minerals and vitamins, work together to help you achieve your maximum energy potential.

Carbohydrates

Carbohydrates are your body's most preferred nutrient. They are also the most maligned. Most of us think of them as the good-tasting treats from Grandma's kitchen that are too tempting to pass up. But they are also found in fruits, beets, onions, carrots, turnips, sweet potatoes, grains, and grain products, such as breakfast cereals, noodles, pastries, and other vegetables.

Carbohydrates are the easiest foods for your body to digest. Aside from providing energy, high-quality carbohydrate foods contain important minerals and vitamins, and ofttimes they come packaged with proteins.

When the carbohydrate stores in your body become inadequate, such as from prolonged, strenuous physical activity or starvation, the body can adjust and allow you to use fats and, infrequently, proteins to fill your energy needs. Unfortunately, the use of fats and proteins in place of carbohydrates is less-efficient and chemically more complex. The use of fats and proteins can continue for only a limited amount of time before other body functions begin to suffer.

Most carbohydrates come in the form of simple sugars or starches. (See Illus. 11-1.) When these carbohydrate foods are eaten, they are digested by your body and broken down into the simple sugars of glucose, fructose, and galactose. These carbohydrates may also be converted to glycogen for future use.

Glycogen is often called animal starch. It is stored in the liver or other tissues such as the muscles, as free or fixed glycogen. The free glycogen is released quickly for food energy whereas the fixed glycogen is released in a slower manner. Glycogen is used up quickly during exercise and starvation. Since most animals cannot store much glycogen, little of it is found in meat.

Cellulose is a carbohydrate but it's harder to digest than starches and sugars. It must be cooked to be digested. Even then, most of the cellulose remains undigested. Cellulose helps elimination by giving bulk to the digestive track. It comes from the seeds, leaves, stems, and roots of fruits.

By learning how carbohydrates are used by your body (see Box 11-1), you'll be better able to understand the information presented in Chapter 12.

There are four important points on this step-by-step description of carbohydrate energy in Box 11-1.

1. Most of our energy from carbohydrates comes in the form of glucose.
2. Galactose and glucose need insulin to get across the cell membrane, fructose does not.
3. Starches are broken down more slowly by the body's digestive system.
4. Fructose is broken down, absorbed, and used more slowly than glucose and galactose.

These four concepts have important implications in energy utilization as will be shown in the next chapter.

Researchers agree that your optimum carbohydrate sources for energy are

Molecular Compositions of Carbohydrates

Simple Sugars (Monosaccharides):

Double Sugars (Disaccharides):

Glucose: plants

Maltose: malted milk, malted breakfast foods, corn syrups, grains

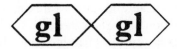

Fructose: fruits

Sucrose: sugar cane, beets, sap sugars

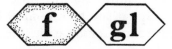

Galactose: milk, milk products

Lactose: milk, milk products

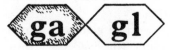

Starches (Polysaccharides): whole grains and whole grain products, beans, peas, and root vegetables, i.e., potatoes

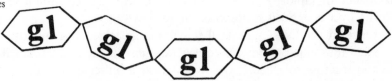

The above would be a small section of the molecule, since a polysaccharide is made up of hundreds of units of sugar.

Illus. 11-1   The simple and double carbohydrates are referred to as sugars, while the multiple ones are called starches. All carbohydrates consist of oxygen, hydrogen, and carbon atoms.

Box 11-1 Summary of the Use of Carbohydrates for Food Energy

Step 1—Carbohydrates are eaten in the form of simple sugars (single or double) and starches. The great majority of your single and double sugars are sucrose (cane or beet sugar), lactose (milk sugar), or fructose (fruit sugar). Most of your starches come from grains and vegetables. Once these sugars and starches are eaten, they move into the stomach for partial digestion, and then into the small intestine.

Step 2—In the small intestine almost all sugars and starches are broken down into the simple sugars of glucose, fructose, and galactose. Approximately 80 percent end up being glucose, 10 percent fructose, and 10 percent galactose. Glucose, fructose, and galactose are released more quickly than the starches since they are already simple sugars. But the starches, too, are broken down into glucose and are released into the bloodstream. Consequently, the starches are eventually reduced to glucose, but their release into the bloodstream is a lot slower.

Step 3—As these three sugars pass out of the small intestine, glucose and galactose move rapidly into the liver's blood system. Fructose, however, moves through the intestine slowly. And as it does, *most* is changed to glucose.

Step 4—The glucose and remaining galactose and fructose must then move into the liver itself. Insulin, along with a small protein molecule, helps to transport the glucose and galactose across the liver cell membrane. (Insulin's job is to speed the galactose and glucose across the liver's cell membrane rapidly.) Fructose does not appear to need insulin to get into the liver cell. So it is absorbed more slowly.

Once in the liver, almost all remaining galactose and fructose are converted into glucose. Besides converting most of the remaining galactose and fructose to glucose, the liver acts as a buffer on blood glucose levels by converting the excess glucose into glycogen for future use or possibly even fat.

Step 5—The glucose and the small remaining amounts of fructose and galactose are released by the liver into the bloodstream and delivered to the cells of the body.

Step 6—To get into the various cells of the body a pattern similar to Step 4 is followed. That is, galactose and glucose are assisted by insulin whereas fructose is not. As an aside, it's important to note that the brain cells are an exception, since insulin is not needed for the glucose to get into the brain.

Once in the cell, the glucose and fructose are used readily for cell function. Any glucose or fructose left over is converted into glycogen. The galactose, however, is released from the cell and sent back to the liver for conversion into glucose.

Step 7—When the cell is completely filled with glycogen, the remaining glucose is sent to the liver and converted into a triglyceride and stored in the fat cells of your body.

---

complex carbohydrates. The least desirable source is sucrose, since it floods the bloodstream with excessive glucose—but more on this later.

These foods (complex carbohydrates) allow for a steady stream of energy. Complex carbohydrates release about two calories of energy per minute. This rate is ideally suited to the needs of your body.

It has been proven that a diet high in carbohydrates will give you more stamina for heavy physical labor than will a diet high in protein, fats, or a combination of protein, fats, and carbohydrates. As far back as 1939, two Scandinavian physiologists, D.H. Christensen and O. Hansen, noted that the composition of a person's diet had a marked influence on how long he was able to continue heavy exercise. Diets rich in carbohydrates improved the exerciser's ability to continue exercising. Diets poor in carbohydrates, however, were associated with a reduced ability to exercise.

Almost 30 years later another group of Scandinavian physiologists determined that the relative composition of an exerciser's diet was closely related to the concentration of glycogen in the muscles. They further noted that exhaustion occurred when the muscle glycogen concentration was very low. Obviously, a carbohydrate-rich diet increases your amount of muscle glycogen. This greater concentration of muscle glycogen delays the time when critically low levels of muscle glycogen are reached. So, the length of time it takes for a person to become physically exhausted when exercising for long periods of time is increased. To go back to the automotive analogy, diets rich in carbohydrates act to increase the capacity of our fuel tanks, thus increasing our cruising range.

This technique of using carbohydrates for more energy is called carbohydrate loading, glycogen packing, or carbohydrate packing. Essentially, in carbohydrate loading the athlete attempts to increase his storage of glycogen before a performance or race. A seven-day regimen of glycogen loading might look like this:

Sunday: Strenuous exercise (depletion of glycogen stores)
Monday: Moderate exercise (very little carbohydrates)
Tuesday: Moderate exercise (very little carbohydrates)
Wednesday: Light exercise (plenty of carbohydrates)
Thursday: Light exercise (plenty of carbohydrates)
Friday: Light exercise (plenty of carbohydrates)
Saturday: Competition

The primary supply of carbohydrates should come from those foods listed in Table 11-1 and you should avoid high amounts of pastry.

Carbohydrate loading causes you to first reduce your glycogen content and then you encourage your body to store an extra amount in the muscles—perhaps 10 percent. Caution should be taken, however, since carbohydrates tend to bind with water and some people experience a rather rapid weight gain (although it is water), and a feeling of sluggishness or of being heavy.

A shorter form of glycogen packing would be as follows:

Tuesday: Strenuous exercise (glycogen depletion)
Wednesday: Light exercise (plenty of carbohydrates)
Thursday: Light exercise (plenty of carbohydrates)
Friday: Light exercise (plenty of carbohydrates)
Saturday: Competition

Just remember this important point: Carbohydrate loading only works with those people who plan to exercise two hours or more. It seems to have little value for the average tennis player, golfer, or jogger. But if you're going to split wood for two or three hours, bike, run a marathon, or work hard physically all day, it's good to know that carbohydrates are your best energy source.

It's important to note that we're suggesting changes in a relative proportion of one's diet during the days proceeding competition. Far too often, carbohydrate loading is interpreted to mean an excuse to go on a dietary binge. But that means trouble. If you overeat these foods you're going to feel like you've just finished a Thanksgiving or Christmas dinner. Don't gorge yourself with cookies, donuts, pizza, and beer. A relatively normal diet with somewhat reduced quantities of meat and dairy products and proportionately increased

TABLE 11-1
Complex Carbohydrates

Fructose

Apples	Figs	Mangoes	Plums
Apricots	Gooseberries	Muskmelons	Pomegranates
Bananas	Grapefruit	Nectarines	Quinces
Blackberries	Grapes	Oranges	Raisins
Blueberries	Guava	Papayas	Raspberries
Breadfruit	Kumquats	Peaches	Strawberries
Cherries	Lemon juice	Pears	Tangerines
Cranberries	Loganberries	Persimmons	Watermelon
Dates	Lychees	Pineapple	

Grains

Barley	Cornmeal	Popcorn	Rye
Buckwheat	Oatmeal	Rice	Wheat

Vegetables

Artichokes	Carrots, raw	Legumes (dried)	Pumpkins
Asparagus	Cauliflower	Lentils	Radishes
Bamboo shoots	Celery	Lettuce	Rutabagas
Bean sprouts	Chives	Mustard greens	Squash
Beans, snap green	Corn kernels	Okra	Sweet potatoes
and yellow	Cucumbers	Onions	Swiss chard
Beans, lima	Eggplant	Parsley	Tapioca
Beans, pinto	Endive	Parsnips	Tomatoes
Beets	Garbanzos	Peas	Turnips
Broccoli	Garlic	Peppers	Water chestnuts
Cabbage, raw	Leeks	Potatoes	

quantities of vegetables, fruits, and bread is best. Foods like ice cream, chocolate, cakes, and crackers contain large amounts of fat and are not necessary in your diet.

Fats

Fats have a bad reputation in our society. Most people think that if they eat fats they'll get fat. But eating a certain amount of fat is essential if you expect to maintain a well-balanced energy diet.

Fats are actually a class of nutrients made up of fatty acids and glycerin (an organic alcohol). They are found in such foods as butter and other dairy products, fatty meats, fish, egg yolks, poultry, salad and cooking oils, margarine, chocolate, nuts, and peanut butter. Pound for pound, fats provide more usable energy than either carbohydrates or proteins. They also take longer to digest so you feel fuller after a meal or a snack that contains some kind of fatty component.

Certain foods contain different chemical compounds, called fats or lipids. These include triglycerides, phospholipids, and cholesterol. The triglycerides are used in the body to provide energy, a function they share with the carbohydrates. The cholesterol and phospholipids, however, are used throughout the body for other cell functions. Consequently, the primary emphasis here will be on triglycerides.

Thirty to 50 percent of all the carbohydrates you eat with each meal are converted into triglycerides in the liver and then stored in the fat cells and later used as fatty acids for energy. Your body can store only small amounts of glycogen (carbohydrates). However, the average person can store up to 200 times as much energy in the form of fat. This difference is important when you think of exercising for long periods of time and engaging in hard physical labor for many weeks.

During very light or moderate muscular exercise—walking, playing pool, sailing, and easy jogging—energy is derived in almost equal amounts from your body's stores of carbohydrates and fats. In an all-out run, however, most of the energy comes from carbohydrates. That's because as the exercise becomes more and more intense, your body produces lactic acid. When lactic acid begins to appear in the blood some fatty acids are blocked, which means that your body must rely on carbohydrates for energy. The more intense the exercise, the more lactic acid; hence, fewer fatty acids are used.

When you exercise at more moderate levels your body works the other way. That is, if you run moderately or swim moderately for an hour or so, there is a significant shift in your body metabolism so that you start using more fatty acids and fewer carbohydrates. If you run for an hour or so, 90 percent of your energy may come from fats and 10 percent from carbohydrates.

This phenomenon of fat-utilization and of lactic acid blocking the fat has important energy implications. People who are unfit produce quite a bit of lactic acid at relatively low levels of exercise. Consequently, they use less fat for energy than do fit people. As they become fit, however, they produce less lactic acid and therefore burn more fat.

The significance of this fat use is that your body contains less carbohydrates than fat, so much so that when you're working for long periods of time, the successful burning of fat helps to spare the carbohydrate—and you experience less fatigue.

Box 11-2 Summary of the Use of Fats for Food Energy

Step 1—Fats eaten (dietary fats) are digested and then released by the digestive system into the lymphatic system. The lymph system literally dumps the fats into the bloodstream.

Step 2—The dietary fats are transported through the small blood vessels of the fat cells. Since the triglyceride molecule is too big to pass through the fat cell membrane, an enzyme reduces the triglyceride into fatty acids and glycerol.

There are three kinds of fatty acids: saturated, unsaturated, and polyunsaturated. These terms refer to the manner in which the hydrogen and carbon atoms of the fat are fastened together. Illustration 11-2 shows the differences in the molecular structure of the three different types of fat.

Step 3—As the fatty acids pass through the fat cells they change back into a triglyceride, which is stored for future use. Eighty to 95 percent of the volume of a fat cell is triglyceride.

Step 4—When the body needs energy, the triglycerides are broken down again and the fatty acid molecules pass into the blood for utilization by the cells.*

Step 5—The way fatty acids are used for energy is complicated. But essentially, when the fatty acid re-enters the cell, the mitochondria of the cell (the powerhouse) uses the fatty acid for food energy, much as glucose is used for food energy.

*Some fatty acids are combined with plasma protein to form lipoproteins. In this manner the fatty acids are delivered to the other cells.

The lipoproteins come in three major forms:

Very Low Density Lipoproteins—These are high in triglycerides and moderately high in phospholipids and cholesterol. The very low density lipoproteins transport the fatty acids (triglycerides) from the liver to the fat tissue.

Low-Density Lipoproteins—When the very low density lipoproteins release the triglycerides they become low-density lipoproteins, consequently they are low in triglycerides and high in cholesterol.

High-Density Lipoproteins—The high-density lipoproteins are 50 percent protein and contain only small amounts of fat. They also probably act as cholesterol scavengers to clear out extra cholesterol from the circulatory system and return it to the liver for excretion.

Three Types of Fat

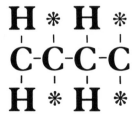

Saturated	Unsaturated	Polyunsaturated
beef	almonds	corn oil
butter	cashews	fish
cheese (whole milk)	chicken	herring oil
chocolate	duck	margarine (nonhydrogenated
coconut	olive oil	soybean oil)
cream	peanuts	safflower oil
eggs	peanut oil	soybean oil
ice cream	pecans	walnuts
lamb	turkey	wheat germ oil
margarines (ordinary)		
milk (whole)		
pork		
shortenings (hydrogenated)		
veal		

Illus. 11-2 In saturated fats each carbon atom has two hydrogen atoms attached. In unsaturated fats one carbon atom is free of hydrogen. The polyunsaturated fats, on the other hand, have two or more carbon atoms free of hydrogen.

The traditional approach to improving energy (as we discussed under carbohydrate energy) has been to attempt to enlarge the total amount of glycogen that the body can store. In other words, your body tries to create a large fuel storage tank. Interestingly, some researchers are also looking at how to spare the rate of glycogen used—how to improve the body's gas mileage. Most studies show that it's probably more important to slow the rate of glycogen release than it is to increase the total size of glycogen stores.

A runner's diet just before a run can have a profound influence upon the rate of glycogen used. Some runners who practice carbohydrate loading believe that extra carbohydrates should be eaten right up to the start of the race. That is not a good idea. Release of insulin into the blood following the eating of carbohydrates acts to block the release of fatty acids from the fat tissue. That means that there is a decrease in the concentration of circulating fatty acids. Consequently, muscle glycogen and blood glucose are the only fuels potentially available for muscular contraction. During exercise, an increased rate of muscle glycogen use occurs and there's a rapid initial drop in blood glucose. If the exercise is continued, fatigue from muscle glycogen depletion occurs at a rate faster than normal. Also, in a few people blood glucose continues to fall until hypoglycemia occurs. Hypoglycemia produces overpowering weariness, light-headedness, irritability, and occasional fainting. Those feelings occur when the blood glucose level falls to a point where the fuel supply to the brain becomes limited.

The unfavorable response to immediate pre-exercise eating appears to be alleviated by the insulin secreted in response to the carbohydrates in a meal. If the meal is eaten far enough in advance to allow complete digestion, the insulin levels will be normal. So the fatty acids are not blocked. In most cases, a meal three to six hours before prolonged exercise will allow adequate deple-tion. Since most long exercise sessions are generally started in the morning, the most practical solution to the prerun feeding problem is to eat your last meal during the evening. That way you'll come to the start of the event with an empty stomach.

For example, let's say you plan a long hike one morning while on vacation. Eat a good, well-balanced meal high in complex carbohydrates the night before. For breakfast, keep it light—perhaps a glass of orange juice and a piece of toast. Carry some fruit along the trail and eat that when you get hungry. Then when you finish your hike, return to your normal eating habits. The key to eating before extended, strenuous exercise is to give your digestive system very little work to do from three to six hours before you begin. That way, you will improve your fuel economy.

Proteins

Proteins are present in all living tissues. They make up vital parts of cells and are the main constituents of muscles, nerves, glands, and many hormones. Protein molecules are large and are composed of many nitrogen-containing components called amino acids. Individual protein molecules may consist of several different amino acids. Before your body can use these proteins they must be broken down into their component amino acids by the digestive system.

There are 21 amino acids, of which your body can manufacture 11. They are called nonessential. The other 10, called essential amino acids, can be obtained only by eating the right foods.

Your body uses proteins to build and repair body tissues, and in emergency situations your body can oxidize proteins to meet energy needs. However, using proteins for energy can go on for only a short period of time, because while proteins are being oxidized for energy the building and repairing process of body cells and tissues comes to a temporary halt. Only proteins can supply the necessary amino acids that your body needs. If your protein supply is not sufficient to offset the daily destruction of cells, your body actually begins to waste away. So a poor protein diet will have serious negative effects on your growth and development.

Proteins are crucial, but they are not required in large amounts. Meat, fish, eggs, and nuts are rich in complete protein. They contain all the essential amino acids. Dry cereals, breads, and most fruits and vegetables contain lesser amounts of proteins. Additionally, these proteins are incomplete, which means that they do not contain all of the ten essential amino acids. They do contain some. These foods are good, but for most effective use by our bodies they should be combined with other protein fats to make them more effective. (See Table 11-2.)

Many of these foods also provide some minerals and vitamins. It's important to get protein from a wide range of sources, particularly during periods of rapid growth and cell formation, as in adolescence, pregnancy, and convalescence. It is a common practice among doctors to prescribe high protein diets for pregnant women and individuals with diseases where there has been a high degree of cell destruction or damage.

These four steps in Box 11-3 explain how proteins are used for energy when there is an excess of protein. But when there is a lack of carbohydrates or fat your body must use protein for energy. Your body uses what protein you have in your diet. Utilization of protein for food energy is far less efficient than using carbohydrates and fats. Because your body prefers carbohydrates and fats for food energy, both are called protein sparers.

Vitamins

Vitamins are not food energy sources per se. That is, they don't provide calories. But vitamins are a very important energy source, making it possible for us to use the food we eat appropriately. They provide for chemical control of your body functions and play an important role in energy production, normal

TABLE 11-2
Protein Foods

Animal Products

Beef	Duck	Fish	Pork
Cheese	Eggs	Milk	Turkey
Chicken			

Grains

Brown Rice	Corn	Oats	Rice

Legumes

Garbanzo Beans	Lima Beans	Peas	Soybean Flour
Kidney Beans	Mung Beans	Soy Sprouts	Soybeans

Nuts and Seeds

Cashews	Peanuts

Vegetarian Dishes*

Barley and yogurt soup
Bean or pea curry on rice
Blended dip of garbanzos, sesame, lemon, garlic, oil
Bread made with milk or cheese
Breads with added seed meals
Breads with sesame or sunflower seed spread
Cereal with milk
Cheese sandwiches
Cheese sauce for garbanzo beans
Corn-soy bread
Corn tortillas and beans
Legume soup with bread
Lentil curry on rice
Macaroni and cheese
Middle Eastern hummus (sesame and chick-peas)
Milk in legume soups
Pasta with milk or cheese
Pea soup and toast
Rice and milk pudding
Rice-bean casserole
Rice-cheese casserole
Rice with sesame seeds
Roasted seeds—soybean snack
Sesame salt on legume dish
Sesame seeds in bean soups and casseroles
Sunflower seeds and peanuts
Wheat berries with cheese sauce
Wheat bread with baked beans
Wheat-soy bread

SOURCE: Based on Frances Lappe's *Diet for a Small Planet* (New York: Ballantine, 1975).
*These dishes show how you can combine nonmeat protein foods (those not containing all ten essential amino acids) to make a complete protein dish.

growth, resistance to infection, and general health. Most vitamins act as catalysts that initiate or speed up the rate of chemical reactions. Life cannot continue without these biochemical catalysts.

Nevertheless, vitamins cannot catalyze anything on their own. They must first combine with substances called apoenzymes, which are manufactured within each individual cell. When a cell is making apoenzymes at its maximum speed, and they are combining with vitamins as fast as they are made, the cell

Box 11-3 Summary of the Use of Proteins for Food Energy

Step 1—There is an upper limit to the amount of protein that can accumulate in each cell. Once the cells are filled, the additional amino acids are sent to the liver.

Step 2—Once in the liver, the 21 amino acids are degraded into glucose, glycogen, or fat for future use.

Step 3—Eighteen of the 21 amino acids have the chemical structure that permits them to be converted into glucose. Nineteen can be converted into fat (5 directly and 14 by being converted into carbohydrates first and then into fat).

Step 4—Once the amino acids are changed into glucose or fat they are used by the body in those forms.

is said to be saturated with that particular vitamin. Once the whole body is saturated, any excess vitamins can't act as vitamins at all. So, like any other chemical or drug you eat, they are stored or circulated in the bloodstream.

Most plants manufacture the vitamins they need. For the most part, your body can't do that. You must get your vitamins from the foods you eat. The highest sources of vitamins are meats, particularly the liver and kidneys; fruits; vegetables; milk; eggs; fish; and certain cereals. Vitamin deficiencies can result in night blindness, poor bone and tooth formation, scurvy, stunted growth, lack of vitality, poor condition of skin and mucous membranes, and a loss of appetite and weight.

Perhaps you've wondered why vitamins are designated by a letter of the alphabet. The reason is because at one time scientists did not know their chemical structure and could not give them proper scientific names. There are two basic kinds of vitamins: water-soluble and fat-soluble. The fat-soluble vitamins are A, D, E, and K. The water-soluble vitamins are vitamin B, in particular B_1 and B_2 and niacin, pyridoxine, B_{12}, folic acid, biotin, and pantothenic acid, and vitamin C.

When many people talk about nutrition they think only of vitamins. They faithfully study the chart on the side of the cereal boxes to see whether they're getting their vitamins. But if you ate nothing but bowls of cereal every day for the rest of your life and nothing else, you probably wouldn't live very long, even if you thought you were getting enough vitamins. That's because you're simply getting vitamins and carbohydrates and not an adequate amount of protein, selected minerals, and other essential vitamins.

There is a tremendous controversy regarding how much vitamins are needed by Americans. On one side of the coin you have the traditional medical establishment, which advocates the United States government recommended daily allowance (RDA) on vitamins. (See Table 11-3.) On the other side of the coin there are a few famous biochemists, Drs. Linus Pauling and Roger Williams, recommending megavitamins. Megavitamins are large doses of certain vitamins to reduce the incidence of disease—everything from the common cold to cancer. When it comes to the role of vitamins in building energy, the scene is even more cloudy. Quite frankly, the vitamin story is far from complete. Researchers just don't know. Their findings have not been definitive. Most of the studies show that supplementing an already well-balanced diet will not produce an increase in energy. But, and it's a big one, most of these studies have been conducted over relatively short periods of time. We don't know what effect vitamin supplementation has over a 10-, 15-, or 20-year period of time.

It's probably an individual kind of thing. I subscribe to what Dr. Williams calls biological individuality. Each person is different. What is appropriate for one person may not be appropriate for another. Even traditional scientists and physicians should accept that fact. After all, they recognize that many forms of medication have to be adjusted for each person, so why couldn't there be a variance with respect to vitamins? The federal government notes that the RDA is not based on just what prevents a deficiency. Instead they try to look at individual differences and add a safety factor above that. Consequently the RDA of vitamin C for adults is 45 milligrams (mg.). Five mg. is supposed to prevent a deficiency, and it takes around 35 to 40 mg. a day to saturate the cells.

Research however, has demonstrated that certain people need extra vitamins. Heavy drinkers, for example, are often deficient in many of the B vitamins. Very heavy drinkers have an even more serious problem. People who drink six or seven drinks a day over a two-week period of time begin to suffer from starvation no matter how much they eat and no matter how well balanced their diet is. Under conditions of alcohol abuse, the small intestine pours out fluids and flushes food from the body before vitamins and minerals can be absorbed.

Heavy smokers also tend to be depleted of vitamin C. Additionally,

TABLE 11-3
U.S. Recommended Daily Allowances (RDA) of Vitamins and Minerals

Key
1 microgram (mcg.) = 1/1000 of a milligram = 1 gamma
1,000 micrograms = 1 milligram (mg.)
1,000 milligrams = 1 gram (g.)
1,000 grams = 1 kilogram (kg.)

Vitamin	U.S. RDA
A	5,000 International Units (IU)
D	200–400 IU (5–10 mcg.)
E	15 IU Men (10 mg.)—12 IU Women (8 mg.)
K	70–140 mcg.
B_1 Thiamine	1.4 mg. Men-1 mg. Women
B_2 Riboflavin	1.6 mg. Men-1.2 mg. Women
B_3 Niacin	18 mg. Men-13 mg. Women
B_5 Pantothenic Acid	4–7 mg.
B_6 Pyridoxine	2.2 mg. Men-2 mg. Women
Biotin	1.3 mg.
Folacin	1.4 mg.
B_{12} Cyanocabalamin	3 mcg.
C	60 mg.

Mineral	U.S. RDA
Calcium	800 mg.
Magnesium	350 mg. Men-300 mg. Women
Phosphorus	800 mg.
Potassium	1,875–5,625 mg.
Sodium	1,100–3,300 mg.
Sulfur	. . .

Trace Mineral	U.S. RDA
Chromium	.05–.2 mg.
Copper	2–3 mg.
Fluorine	. . .
Iodine	150 mcg.
Iron	18 mg.
Manganese	2.5–5 mg.
Selenium	. . .
Zinc	15 mg.

women who are using a birth control pill seem to have difficulty securing enough of the B vitamins and vitamin C.

We cannot assume that if a little of a vitamin is good for you, a lot is even better. When your cells are vitamin saturated, additional vitamins are worthless. Consequently, I recommend experimentation. In Table 11-4 I've given you information on vitamins and their potential relationship to building energy. Please note that I have listed the RDA from the federal government. You need that much. Also listed are what the megavitamin people have suggested. Finally, information is provided regarding the proven role of vitamins in the body as well as the speculative roles that have been bandied about by vitamin enthusiasts. I've also tried to indicate some potential harmful effects of too much of selected vitamins.

My own recommendation is to make sure that you get your RDA. If you are having some of the problems listed under the known role of vitamins in the body, or are showing signs of deficiency, then you could try taking additional amounts of the vitamin. If you decide to go to the megadoses I would suggest that you discuss this with your physician. (Note: I also suggest that you get as many of your vitamins as possible from fresh fruits and vegetables. Avoid canned vegetables and fruits. They have a greatly reduced vitamin and mineral content. Eating most fruits and vegetables raw or steamed is best. If you must cook them, cook lightly and try to save the juice. Also choose whole grain breads and cereals rather than refined ones, and select brown rice instead of white. Finally, eat a wide variety of foods. As for meat, try some seafood and fowl in place of pork and beef.

Minerals

Minerals are unique, inorganic chemical substances. Like vitamins, they play an important part in regulating body functions and are essential to the structure of bones and other body tissues. They are vital to your energy.

Minerals are part of the cell membrane, cell nucleus, and other cell structures—such as the mitochondria, or powerhouses of the cell. This powerhouse converts food nutrients to energy. For example, selected minerals help break down glucose, fatty acids, and amino acids into energy. All other minerals build up the glucose, fatty acids, and amino acids into glycogen, fats, and proteins respectively. Minerals also serve as important parts of the structure of various hormones, enzymes, and other substances that help to regulate the chemical reactions within cells.

Text Continues on Page 160

TABLE 11-4
Vitamins and
Their Relationship to Building Energy

Fat-Soluble Vitamins/Those Most Likely to Be Deficient	Energy Role	Sources	U.S. RDA	Mega-vitamin Recommendations
A College students, cigarette smokers, drug users, marijuana smokers, alcoholics, nursing mothers, and people living in polluted areas.	Plays a role in formation of the hormone cortisone.	Carrots, peas, lettuce, sweet potatoes, tomatoes, liver, eggs, dairy foods, apricots, fresh fruits, squash, cantaloupe, butter, fortified margarine, and broccoli.	5,000 International Units(IU)	10,000 to 35,000 IU
D People with colds or the flu, pregnant women, and heart disease patients.	Unknown.	Sunlight, fish, liver, oils, and fortified milk. Small amounts are found in butter, liver, and egg yolk.	400 IU	400 to 1,000 IU
E People who are exposed to air pollution, people who eat refined white flour, highly stressed individuals, diabetics, pregnant and lactating women, the aged, people using birth control pills, and heart disease patients.	Protects fat in the body's tissue from an abnormal breakdown.	Vegetable oils—cottonseed, safflower, sunflower, soybean; corn, almonds, peanuts, whole grains, wheat germ, nuts, legumes, eggs, and sprouts.	15 IU Men 12 IU Women	200 to 800 IU

Known Health Roles	Unproven But Possible Roles in the Body	Deficiency Signs	Toxic Effect
Vitamin A is important in the formation of the mucous membranes and skin. It helps in preventing eye disorders. It's also important in bone and teeth formation.	May be important for tissue health and preventing precancer cells from becoming cancerous. There is also some evidence that vitamin A may play a role in prevention of colds and other viral infections.	Stunting of growth, impairment of vision, diseased conditions of the skin and membranes lining the respiratory passages and digestive and genital-urinary tracts, and abnormalities in enamel-forming cells of teeth.	Excessive irritability, dry itchy skin, headaches, nausea, and diarrhea. Yellowing of the skin and eye whites, painful joint swellings. Fragile bones and enlarged liver and spleen. Deaths have been reported.
It's needed during periods of growth for bones and teeth, and required throughout life for calcium metabolism.	Unknown.	Weight loss, loss of appetite, cramps, poor bone formation, and rickets.	Unusual thirst, urinary urgency, vomiting, and diarrhea.
Acts as an antioxidant to reduce oxidation of vitamin A and polyunsaturated fatty acids.	May be involved in the aging process, slowing down heart disease, and reducing incidence of cancer.	Pigmentation and anemia.	Unknown.

Table 11-4—Continued

Fat-Soluble Vitamins/Those Most Likely to Be Deficient	Energy Role	Sources	U.S. RDA	Mega-vitamin Recom-menda-tions
K People who take aspirin, antibiotic users, people on anticoagulants, those living in polluted environments, people who eat lots of frozen foods, patients recovering from surgery, and the aged.	Unknown.	Lettuce, spinach, kale, cauliflower, cabbage, other leafy, green vegetables, liver, egg yolk, and soybean.	70–140 micro-grams (mcg.)	Unknown.
Water-Soluble Vitamins/Those Most Likely to Be Deficient	**Energy Role**	**Sources**	**U.S. RDA**	**Mega-vitamin Recom-menda-tions**
B$_1$ Thiamine College students, cigarette smokers, drinkers, pregnant women, heavily stressed individuals, those who do not eat regularly, arthritics, and those who eat white breads and refined white pastries.	Necessary for carbohydrate metabolism and a properly functioning nervous system.	Meat, fish, poultry, eggs, whole grain breads, and cereal. Soybeans, beans, split peas, pork, oatmeal, yeast, wheat germ, sunflower and sesame seeds, and nuts like peanuts.	1.4 milligrams (mg.) Men 1 mg. Women	10 to 100 mg.
B$_2$ Riboflavin College students, those who do not eat regularly, those who are depressed or highly stressed, the aged, and those using oral contraceptives.	Necessary for fat and carbohydrate metabolism.	Milk, cheese, liver kidneys, fish, poultry, eggs, whole grain breads and cereals, cottage cheese, oysters, beef, leafy vegetables, beans, and peas.	1.6 mg. Men 1.2 mg. Women	10 to 100 mg.

Known Health Roles	Unproven But Possible Roles in the Body	Deficiency Signs	Toxic Effect
Necessary for proper blood clotting.	Unknown.	Prolonged clotting time.	Jaundice in children.

Known Health Roles	Unproven But Possible Roles in the Body	Deficiency Signs	Toxic Effect
Thiamine is important in regulating your appetite.	May improve mental processes.	Fatigue, insomnia, irritability, loss of appetite, constipation. Heart irregularity disturbances, digestive balances, muscle tenderness, weight loss, forgetfulness, lassitude, and mental inadequacy are all possibilities. Gross deficiency results in beriberi, a fatal heart disease.	None. Repeated injections of B_1 have caused loss of effectiveness. Occasionally urine may yellow but this is normal. Heart palpitations.
In enzymes that transport hydrogen as part of the metabolism of protein.	May improve mental processes.	Irritation and cracks at corners of the mouth. Scaly skin around nose and ears. Some tongue and mouth itching and burning eyes. Eyes sensitive to light.	None.

Table 11-4—Continued

Water-Soluble Vitamins/Those Most Likely to Be Deficient	Energy Role	Sources	U.S. RDA	Mega-vitamin Recommendations
B₃ Niacin College students, highly stressed individuals, heavy sugar users, hypoglycemics, users of antibiotics, and those eating large amounts of pastries and starches.	Necessary for carbohydrate metabolism.	Meat, liver, fish, poultry, eggs, whole grain breads and cereals, wheat germ, nuts, seeds, rice, beans, and peas.	18 mg. Men 13 mg. Women	50 mg. to 3 grams (g.)
B₅ Pantothenic Acid College students, heavy sugar users, hypoglemics, users of antibiotics, those under emotional stress, arthritics, workers in cold climates, and those eating refined flour products.	Involved in release of energy from fat and carbohydrates. Used in adrenal gland function and is necessary to fight stress.	Whole grain cereals, legumes, animal meats, eggs, wheat germ, peanuts, and peas.	4–7 mg.	10 to 100 mg.
B₆ Pyridoxine College students, dieters, highly stressed individuals, pregnant women, lactating women, heart disease patients, the aged, and alcoholics.	Involved in fat and carbohydrate metabolism.	Liver, ham, lima beans, corn, sunflower seeds, wheat germ, bran, whole grain bread, flour and cereals, potatoes, and brown rice.	2.2 mg. Men 2 mg. Women	10 to 100 mg.
Biotin People with infections.	Energy release.	Liver, yeast, egg yolk, whole grains, nuts, and legumes.	1.3 mg.	10 to 75 mg.

Known Health Roles	Unproven But Possible Roles in the Body	Deficiency Signs	Toxic Effect
Function is related to protein metabolism.	May help to cure some mental disturbances.	Loss of appetite, nervousness, mental depression, soreness and redness of the tongue, skin pigmentation, ulceration of the gums, and diarrhea. Gross deficiency causes pellagra.	Heart palpitations. Do not use megavitamin doses if you have severe diabetes, cirrhosis of the liver, peptic ulcer, or glaucoma.
See Energy Role.	Some scientists have speculated that it may help the body to utilize cholesterol more effectively and to help in the treatment of arthritis.	A deficiency is rarely seen unless your diet consists of highly processed food. Sore tongue, weakness, weight loss, headache, fatigue, and muscle cramps are common.	None.
Protein metabolism and health of central nervous system.	Causes better handling of cholesterol by the body and it may be helpful with arthritis.	Loss of appetite, diarrhea, skin and mouth disorders, and blindness.	None, but urine may turn yellow. Possible heart palpitations.
Biotin is important in cellular metabolism and helps in the metabolism of fats, carbohydrates, and proteins.	It may help prevent heart disease.	Anemia, muscular pain, and skin disorders. Rare —eating a balanced diet provides 150–300 g. daily. Some drugs such as antibiotics may destroy your body's own ability to synthesize biotin.	Unknown.

Table 11-4—Continued

Water-Soluble Vitamins/Those Most Likely to Be Deficient	Energy Role	Sources	U.S. RDA	Mega-vitamin Recommendations
Folacin Highly stressed individuals, alcoholics, diabetics, those using sulfa drugs, pregnant women, women who experience excessive menstruation, and the aged.	Formation of red blood cells.	Green, leafy vegetables, eggs, liver, kidneys, wheat germ, and yeast.	1.4 mg.	Not recommended, may mask pernicious anemia.
B$_{12}$ Cyanocobalamin Vegetarians, people suffering from irregular menstruation, frequent laxative users, and the aged.	Red blood cell formation.	Present only in animal tissues. That is meats, poultry, fish, shellfish, eggs, and milk products.	3 (mcg.)	5 to 100 mcg.
C Alcoholics, cigarette smokers, college students, users of antibiotics, people taking large amounts of aspirin, heroin addicts, and the aged.	May be important in the healing process and red blood cell formation. Is needed by the adrenal glands to fight stress.	Citrus fruits, tomatoes, strawberries, cranberries, potatoes, raw greens, peppers, broccoli, and cauliflower.	60 mg.	500 mg. to 4 g.

For years nutritionists have emphasized the major minerals. They are calcium, magnesium, phosphorus, potassium, sodium, and sulfur. These have been considered the essential nutrients. Table 11-5 gives you an idea of the role and sources of these particular important elements.

More recently the trace elements or minerals have been brought into the fore. Work begun by Dr. Henry A. Schroeder, professor emeritus at Dartmouth Medical School, has demonstrated that trace elements, although present in minute amounts, are essential for normal metabolism. They include chromium, copper, fluorine, iodine, iron, manganese, selenium, zinc, and a few others.

According to Schroeder's thesis, unlike vitamins, which are synthesized by

Known Health Roles	Unproven But Possible Roles in the Body	Deficiency Signs	Toxic Effect
Assists in formation of certain body proteins.	Unknown.	Smooth red tongue, intestinal upsets, diarrhea, macrocytic anemia. Young red blood cells do not mature.	None.
See Energy Role.	It may also be involved in nucleic acid action and related to nucleic acid therapy in aging.	Anemia, tingling of hands and feet, back pain, mental and nervous change.	Heart palpitations.
Necessary for helping to hold the cells together including in the bones, teeth, skin, organs, and capillary walls.	May help in reducing severity of cold symptoms. May also have some relationship to cholesterol deposits and prevention of cancer. May be involved in metabolism of carbohydrates.	Bleeding and receding gums, unexpected bruises, slow healing, and scurvy.	No known signs other than frequent urination and diarrhea.

plants and animals, minerals—of equal or even greater importance—must come from the outside, and failing to provide them in our diets can lead to trouble.

Schroeder notes that those elements that occur in amounts less than 0.01 percent of the human body are trace elements. While this definition is narrow and restrictive, research demonstrates that they are important for our health and maximum personal energy. Table 11-6 demonstrates the effect of these trace minerals in building energy and vitality.

TABLE 11-5
Minerals and
Their Relationship to Building Energy

Minerals/Those Most Likely to Be Deficient	Energy Role	Sources	U.S. RDA
Calcium People taking large amounts of vitamin A, C, and D; heavy chocolate eaters; inactive and sedentary people; highly stressed individuals; people over 50 years of age, arthritics, people taking laxatives, and heavy water drinkers.	Unknown.	Milk, dark green, leafy vegetables, small fish eaten with bones, all cheeses, dried beans and peas, broccoli, artichokes, and sesame seeds.	800 milligrams (mg.)
Magnesium People who are on an unbalanced diet, such as a high cholesterol diet, high sugar diet, or a diet rich in meat, diabetics; those using diuretics; alcoholics; or those exposed to high levels of noise.	Activates enzymes and carbohydrate metabolism in release of energy. Involved in nerve transmission and muscle contraction.	Whole grains, nuts, beans, green leafy vegetables. Processing may result in high losses of magnesium.	350 mg. Men 300 mg. Women
Phosphorus Pregnant women, growing children, adolescents, cancer patients, arthritics, people with high levels of mental stress, significant tooth decay, and people who use a lot of laxatives or antacids.	For metabolism of carbohydrates and fats.	Organ meats, meats, fish, poultry, eggs, milk, cheese, nuts, beans, peas, and whole grains.	800 mg.

Known Health Roles	Unproven But Possible Roles in the Body	Deficiency Signs	Toxic Effect
It is necessary for hard bones and teeth, muscle contractions—especially normal heart rhythm, transmission of nerve impulses, proper blood clotting, and to activate a number of enzymes.	Unknown.	In children: stunted growth, retarded bone mineralization, poor bones and teeth, skeletal malformation (rickets). In adults: osteoporosis—brittle porous bones, resulting from demineralization.	May contribute to kidney stones, high levels of calcium in blood and urine, and deposition in soft tissues.
Helps regulate body temperatures and protein synthesis.	Unknown.	Usually seen only in alcoholism when people are on a limited diet of highly processed foods. Weakness, tremors, dizziness, spasms, convulsions, delirium, and depression.	None.
Necessary (with calcium) to form and strengthen bones as part of the nucleic acids.	Unknown.	Seldom seen in humans eating a normal diet. Weakness, bone pain, loss of minerals —especially calcium from bones—poor growth.	None known.

Table 11-5—Continued

Minerals/Those Most Likely to Be Deficient	Energy Role	Sources	U.S. RDA
Potassium People who use diuretics and laxatives, cortisone medication, excessive salt and excessive coffee. Also people suffering from migraine headaches, extreme stress, high blood pressure, hypoglycemia, diarrhea, or alcoholism.	Regulates muscle contractions and heart rhythm. Important in glucose formation.	Fruits, dates, bananas, oranges, cantalopes, tomatoes, vegetables, especially dark green leafy vegetables, liver, meat, fish, poultry, and milk.	1,8765– 5,625 mg.
Sodium Those using diuretics, or who work in a hot, humid environment. Also those who have diarrhea.	Regulates muscle contractions.	Salt, salted foods, monosodium glutamate, soy sauce, baking powder, cheese, milk, shellfish, meat, fish, poultry, eggs, most packaged products.	1,100– 3,300 mg.
Sulfur Vegetarians, people suffering from inadequate protein intake, psoriasis or eczema.	Unknown.	Eggs, meat, milk, cheese, nuts, and legumes.	Unknown.

TABLE 11-6

Trace Minerals and Their Relationship to Building Energy

Trace Minerals/Those Most Likely to Be Deficient	Energy Role	Sources	U.S. RDA
Chromium Diabetics, hypoglycemics, the aged, people who sweat a great deal, vomit, or eat lots of sugar.	Metabolism of glucose and combining of fatty acids and insulin metabolism.	Corn oil, meats, and whole grains.	.05–.2 milligrams (mg.)

Known Health Roles	Unproven But Possible Roles in the Body	Deficiency Signs	Toxic Effect
Major constituent of fluid inside cells. Along with sodium it regulates water balance and nerve transmission. Necessary for protein synthesis	Unknown.	Muscle weakness, nausea, depletion of glycogen, rapid heart beat, and heart failure.	Unknown.
Major constituent of fluid outside the cells, regulates water balance and nerve irritability.	Unknown.	Rare: nausea, diarrhea, abdominal and muscle cramps.	Probably a factor in high blood pressure; certainly a low sodium diet is essential to reduce blood pressure.
Part of proteins, especially in hair, nails, and cartilage. Part of the B vitamin thiamine and biotin. Takes part in detoxification reactions.	Unknown.	None found. A diet adequate in protein (several amino acids contain sulfur) will meet needs.	None known.

Known Health Roles	Unproven But Possible Role in the Body	Deficiency Signs	Toxic Effect
Metabolism of protein and synthesis of cholesterol.	Unknown.	Poor utilization of glucose.	Unknown.

Table 11-6—Continued

Trace Minerals/Those Most Likely to Be Deficient	Energy Role	Sources	U.S. RDA
Copper People who have suffered heavy loss of blood, are anemic, and have a low red blood cell count.	Acts with iron to bind hemoglobin in red blood cells. Necessary for glucose metabolism.	Most foods including organ meats, shellfish, nuts, dried beans, peas, and cocoa. It is absent in dairy products. Copper is found in most unprocessed foods.	2–3 mg.
Fluorine Pregnant women, the aged, and people with dental carries.	Unknown.	Water which is naturally or artificially fluoridated.	Unknown.
Iodine People who perspire a great deal, eat an excessive amount of raw cabbage or cauliflower, or live in an area where the soil is depleted.	Important component of thyroid hormones, helps regular basal metabolism.	Seafood, vegetables grown near the ocean where soil is rich in iodine. Butter, milk, cheese, and eggs if the animal's food has been rich in iodine. Iodized salt is another source.	150 micro-grams (mg.)
Iron Women during menstruation, pregnant women, people who eat low amounts of Vitamin C, have lost blood, experienced rapid growth, or have peptic ulcers.	Carries and transfers oxygen in the blood and tissues.	Liver, meat products, egg yolk, fish, green, leafy vegetables, peas, beans, dried fruit, whole grain cereals, and foods prepared from iron-enriched cereal products.	18 mg.
Manganese Lactating women; the aged; diabetics; and people who eat lots of sugar and sugar products, refined flour products, or few vegetables.	Necessary to use glucose and fats for muscle contractions.	Found in most foods, both plant and animal. Whole grains, legumes, and nuts are good sources.	2.5–5 mg.
Selenium Cigarette smokers, and those living in areas of high air pollution.	Unknown.	Bran, whole grain cereals, broccoli, nuts, onions, tomatoes, and turnips.	Unknown.

Known Health Roles	Unproven But Possible Role in the Body	Deficiency Signs	Toxic Effect
Very important in the first few months of life. Important for nourishment of nerve wall and connective tissue.	May aid healing.	Causes anemia in children. Unknown in adults.	Can result in uremia, heart defects, and hypertension.
Prevention of solid tooth formation and decrease in dental cavities.	Unknown.	Tooth decay in young children. Possibly osteoporosis in adults.	Mottling of tooth enamel, deformed teeth and bones.
Influences growth, mental development, and depositing of protein and fat in the body.	May help prevent mental retardation.	Excess may depress thyroid activity and cause goiter.	Unknown.
Part of the hemoglobin in the blood, myoglobin in the muscles, parts of the cells, the cell nuclei, and many enzymes in the tissues.	Unknown.	Digestion problems, cell damage, anemia. Excess skin pigmentation, lowered ability to handle glucose, cirrhosis of the liver.	Unknown.
Necessary to unite complex carbohydrates, fats, and cholesterol. Important for proper development of bones and the pancreas and tendon structure.	May aid healing.	Rarely seen.	Unknown.
Appears to have a sparing action on vitamin E.	May prevent cancers to digestive tract and destroys fats in tiny blood vessels.	Fatigue.	Unknown.

Table 11-6—Continued

Trace Minerals/Those Most Likely to Be Deficient	Energy Role	Sources	U.S. RDA
Zinc Alcoholics, diabetics, pregnant women, men with prostate trouble, women taking oral contraceptives, those under a high amount of stress, and those on an unbalanced diet.	Important part of the enzymes which move carbon dioxide via red blood cells from the tissues to the lungs. Important in insulin formation.	Wheat germ and bran, whole grains, dried beans and peas, nuts, lean meats, fish, and poultry.	15 mg.

Known Health Roles	Unproven But Possible Role in the Body	Deficiency Signs	Toxic Effect
Important in digestion, protein metabolism, and synthesis of nucleic acids.	May prevent prostate cancer and sterility. May also reduce cholesterol deposits.	Rare in the United States. Can cause retarded growth, retarded sexual development, anemia, and poor healing of wounds.	Nausea, vomiting, diarrhea, and fever.

CHAPTER 12
The Energy Robbers

Just as there are foods that give you energy, there are also foods that rob you of energy. These foods have the potential to undo some or all of the good expected from the energy givers. Classically, nutritionists have called the energy robbers "junk foods." These foods are high in calories and low in nutrients. They contain excessive amounts of one or more of the following constituents: sugar, fat, salt, and caffeine.

Your body has an amazing ability to tolerate a lot of abuse. It will make many adjustments to help you survive and maintain homeostasis—that is, the balance within the body to maintain health and life. Your body is tough and adaptable. But when people consume too much sugar, fats, salt, and caffeine, as many Americans do, personal energy levels decline. As much as you don't want to admit it, you can't have maximum personal energy while living on french fries, doughnuts, hamburgers, cokes, milkshakes, and other deep-fried concoctions from your local greasy spoon. Candy, coffee, pretzels, crackers, cakes, and cream-filled "goodies" are all "baddies" for your energy.

I know what you might be thinking: runners like Bill Rogers, who has won both the Boston and New York Marathons, literally pig down on coffee, soda, candy bars, doughnuts, ice cream, and mayonnaise. Yet they have energy to burn. First, let's understand one very important fact. People like Bill Rogers are special biologically. You cannot compare yourself to them. While they might be able to get away with a certain pattern of eating, it does not logically follow that you can do the same thing—unless you have been blessed with their physical qualities and attributes.

Second, if it were possible for Bill Rogers to compete against himself—

that is, one Bill Rogers on a good diet versus one Bill Rogers on a bad diet—I'd put my money on the good-eating Rogers.

Third, most premier marathoners are in their late twenties and early thirties. Many people don't feel tired at this point in their life. It's usually after eating a jitterbug diet for 30 years that people *start* to fall apart and feel tired.

Fourth, marathoners do follow several other high-energy living patterns. They run, stretch, practice relaxation techniques, are nonsmokers, and use few drugs. As a result, they don't feel the energy drain until later in life.

You simply can't cozy up to junk foods and still achieve your maximum personal energy. There are many reasons why. To start with, let's take a look at sugar, a major "junk" ingredient, to see how it saps energy.

Sugar

While "just a spoonful of sugar" may not harm your energy levels, eating 100 to 120 pounds a year (as the average American does) is energy suicide. That's the entire sugar jar or 20 teaspoons a day. To compound the problem, the average American eats only 5 pounds of fruit, vegetables, and cereal products for every pound of sugar. In 1909, the average was 10 pounds of the wholesome stuff for every pound of sugar. Sugar may give you a temporary lift, but later in the day and over the long haul, it's counter-productive to your energy level.

One of the most frustrating experiences that I have is dealing with young children and energy. Their fifth through fifteenth years are their most vigorous and vital. So it's difficult to explain to them why they should be opting for a lifestyle that builds maximum personal energy. They already have it. Little do they realize that when they reach the age of 20, everything starts to go downhill. And it rapidly accelerates from the thirtieth year on.

Sucrose is ultimately broken down into glucose and fructose for energy. As glucose, it gets into your bloodstream very quickly and then requires insulin to get into your cells. The speed of digestion, the insulin requirement, and the amount of sugar eaten by the average American causes a severe lack of energy for reasons I am about to explain.

Speed of Digestion and Insulin Reaction

Your body's blood sugar level is monitored by both the hypothalamus in the brain and the pancreas. When the blood sugar level falls too low (usually if you haven't eaten for several hours), glucose is released from the liver and/or the fat stores are activated. When your blood sugar level goes too high, insulin is secreted by the pancreas to help speed the glucose into the cells and, thereby, reduces the blood glucose levels.

Certain people, however, seem to have difficulty in handling single sugars well—especially large quantities of single sugars. These individuals experience varying degrees of fatigue, blurred vision, a drunken gait, slurred speech, nausea, sudden changes in mood such as depression, crying, and hostility.

Scientists have not been able to pinpoint the exact cause for this condition. In fact, some doctors don't believe the condition exists. They think it is a figment of their patient's imagination. However, I feel the fatigue may be caused by hypoglycemia or hyperosmolality. Work done by Dr. William J. Hudspeth, associate professor, Department of Psychiatry and Behavioral Science at the University of Nevada School of Medicine in Reno, demonstrated these potential problems quite nicely. His research also demonstrates why some doctors have missed the diagnosis of sugar metabolism problems.

In hypoglycemia too much insulin is secreted, forcing an excessive amount of glucose into the cells and, thereby, reducing blood glucose levels to very low levels. The result is fatigue, depression, dizziness. This condition is easy to recognize since the patient will have low blood sugar levels.

Yet there are some patients who demonstrate these same symptoms but do not have low blood sugar levels. Their condition may be hyperosmolality. In hyperosmolality an excessive amount of insulin is secreted, wreaking havoc on the body. And the one part that seems most affected by the insulin is your brain. According to Hudspeth, "Too much insulin can cause brain cells to absorb more than the usual number of electrolytes (ions that circulate in the blood) and to swell with water." Consequently, the patient exhibits characteristics similar to hypoglycemia. This condition, however, can only be detected by the glucose tolerance test, EEGs (brain wave patterns), and actual glucose and insulin levels. That's why some doctors have missed the patient's problem. Blood sugar levels will not reveal this problem. These additional tests are needed for a definite diagnosis.

The bottom line is that fatigue can be caused by a poor diet. For some people the problem may be too much blood sugar, for others it may be too much insulin, but for both the cause is the same—eating too much sugar.

The treatment for both conditions is also the same. According to Hudspeth, "Keep excessive insulin reactions down by sticking to a diet that is low in refined carbohydrates (natural sources are all right) and low in protein and by reducing stress."

Athletes must also be very much aware of the sugar/insulin reaction. Dr. David Costill of Ball State University's Human Performance Laboratory has noted that insulin accelerates the removal of glucose from the blood. Exercise does the same thing—even if insulin is absent. Therefore, when athletes eat a lot of sugar at the start of a race or before the event, they are headed for trouble. The combination of high insulin secretion and the muscular activity of running causes the glucose to be removed from the blood at a rate faster than either the intestines or the liver can handle efficiently. Consequently, blood glucose levels may fall from the usual levels of 90 to 110 mg. per 100 millimeters (ml.) of blood to 35 mg. per 100 ml. of blood in the first 10 minutes of exercise. The result is that the exerciser's muscles are suddenly deprived of their most important source of fuel—blood glucose. So the body must rely on its next most important source—muscle glycogen. Glycogen is not turned over nearly as quickly as glucose and so, performance is significantly impaired. Research done by Costill working with runners showed that runners fatigued earlier and found running much more difficult when they took a sugar drink 30 to 45 minutes before the exercise session.

Some people may wonder why I condemn sugar so strongly. After all, it's usually billed as an energy builder, or as a food to give you a lift. Table sugar does give you a temporary lift, but only for about 20 minutes. Then the insulin swings into action and the insulin/sugar reaction of lessened energy occurs.

Everything I've talked about up to this point focuses on sucrose. Little is known about what happens when a person eats large amounts of milk or fruit sugar—lactose or fructose. Fructose may be somewhat better than sucrose since it is absorbed more slowly from the gut and does not need insulin to pass into the cells. Consequently, blood sugar may not drop as fast. The same is true of honey, which is high in fructose. Since fructose breaks down slowly during metabolism, it does not overload the pancreas and cause it to release more insulin.

At this stage of the game, scientists don't know if large amounts of other simple sugars cause the same problem—energy-wise—as sucrose. My guess is that if you would eat refined fructose, and the others as you do sucrose—100 plus pounds per year—you would be in the same bind; receiving a lift with a let-down. You must remember that the key reason you don't eat that much fructose is because of the way fructose is delivered to you. You can only eat so many apples before you fill your stomach, and stop eating.

As you will recall from the previous chapter, I also mentioned that the complex carbohydrates are absorbed more slowly from the gut and are released into the bloodstream at about two calories per minute. This steady stream of energy is perfect for your body. Consequently, if you are going to eat before strenuous exercise, it would be far better to eat a diet high in complex carbohydrates rather than simple sugars. Fructose may also be a satisfactory replacement.

The Amount Eaten

The problem with sugar (or sucrose) is the amount eaten, rather than sucrose itself. If you were to eat only a few pounds of sugar a year, or a fraction of an ounce a day, the above discussion would not apply. But since the average American eats about 2 to 2½ pounds of sugar a week, this comes out to 500 to 750 calories a day of pure sugar. This is too much. It amounts to ⅕ to ¼ of your total calories.

This is particularly serious because a diet that is high in sucrose usually tends to be low in other basic nutrients—especially the B vitamins and several essential minerals. Usually the sugar comes highly refined and stripped of any potential of giving a positive contribution to your energy.

Your best diet is one with a lot of natural vegetables and grain products (complex carbohydrates) and small amounts of simple sugars.

Fats

Fats can be a source of energy, but like everything else in this book, they are a double-edged sword. Too much can cause problems.

According to many scientists, fats can rob you of energy for several reasons. First, fats can actually suffocate your tissues by depriving them of oxygen. Both saturated and unsaturated fats form a fatty film around the red blood cells and platelets in your blood. This film causes the cells and platelets to stick together. This is called sludging. Sludging causes the red blood cells to carry less oxygen and makes it more likely that they will plug your tiny blood vessels (capillaries). Because the capillaries get blocked, the watery part of the blood is forced through the capillary walls causing edema—which reduces the amount of oxygen available to the cells. Some experts say that plugging in this manner can cause 5 to 20 percent of your body tissue to be affected. Smoking after a heavy, fat meal compounds the problem. The carbon monoxide in the smoke crowds out the oxygen even more, hence less oxygen gets to the tissues.

Second, a diet high in fat may raise cholesterol levels. This cholesterol tends to deposit on the lining of the arteries. When these linings are occluded, less oxygen gets to the heart and you become a prime candidate for heart disease.

Third, fats rob your energy in the condition of ketosis. A high-fat, high-protein, low-carbohydrate diet is often used to achieve weight loss. Many dieters have found that they are completely wacked out on this diet. They develop unbelievable fatigue. Since their diet is largely fat, the sugar in the blood is burned off rapidly. This forces the body to depend on fat reserves for energy. The fatty acids derived from the fat reserve burn inefficiently. As a result, they produce acid metabolites called ketones. Doctors call this ketone increase ketosis.

Ketosis means that your metabolism resembles that of a diabetic. It is a dangerous condition because the brain is partially starved by the absence of glucose. Glucose is the brain's only source of food, and fatty acids cannot be converted to glucose. A highly acid blood also makes it hard for the body and brain to function properly. Furthermore, ketones are acidic. They may actually change your blood pH. A change in blood pH will produce tremendous fatigue, since a fine balance must be kept. If the blood becomes acidic enough, you can go into ketosis shock, which is often fatal.

Finally, it has been shown that an excessive amount of fatty acids in the bloodstream can cause irregular heart beats and can possibly present problems for the liver.

The conclusion: a high-protein, high-fat, low-carbohydrate diet causes the dieter to be whipped most of the time. My advice: avoid it.

Salt

When we discuss salt, we need to make the distinction between sodium and sodium chloride. Sodium is a trace mineral found naturally in many foods. Your body needs regular, small amounts of sodium. Sodium chloride is a chemically manufactured salt commonly referred to as table salt.

Americans eat more table salt than their bodies need. It has been estimated that the average person probably needs no more than a gram a day. Yet, many Americans eat between 8 and 15 grams per day. We plaster it over pretzels, popcorn, peanuts, potato chips, and french fries. We sprinkle it liberally over mashed potatoes, gravy, meat, and vegetables. Some people even sprinkle salt on fresh apples, grapefruit, and watermelon. We do this because we have been led to believe that salt makes everything taste better. But it doesn't. Salt has a taste of its own. People are enjoying the taste of the table salt, not the fruit, vegetable, or meat. Yet, the typical American palate responds to any and all foods with one four-word phrase, "It needs more salt."

Unfortunately, table salt may be a precipitator of hypertension or high blood pressure in many Americans. High blood pressure is one of the biggest causes for fatigue in this country. So, if you have fatigue and don't know what your blood pressure is, I suggest that you have your doctor check it out for you. High blood pressure may cause fatigue because of a feedback mechanism. When your blood pressure rises, your body interprets it as your needing rest to drop the pressure. So, selected receptors signal you to be tired. When you rest, your blood pressure then drops.

The salt/high blood pressure issue is subject to debate. There are some cardiologists who claim that if we eliminated salt from the American diet there would be absolutely no high blood pressure in the U.S.A. There are other experts who claim that the jury is still out. But one thing is clear, cultures around the world that eat little salt—Eskimos, Australians, Aborigines, and Panamanian Indians—have very low rates of high blood pressure, while people like the Northern Japanese, who eat 35 or more grams of salt a day have unbelievably high rates of hypertension—four persons out of ten. Also, when people eat a diet low in salt after having high blood pressure, the high blood pressure usually drops drastically.

Why does table salt seem to cause high blood pressure? No one is sure, but there are several plausible explanations. The extra salt eaten causes more fluid to be retained. When you retain fluid between the tissues, this makes it more difficult for the blood to flow through the tiny blood vessels. Since these small blood vessels are somewhat blocked by the pressure put on them, the blood has a more difficult time getting through. This raises the blood pressure. When a person drops his salt intake, he loses not only salt in his body but water as well. The loss of water reduces the pressure on the tiny capillaries, hence the blood can get through. The result is a lower blood pressure.

Since table salt also forces the body to retain fluids, extra salt can cause a weight gain. The weight is not due to fat but water. Extra pounds due to water is like extra weight due to an excessive amount of fat. It causes early fatigue, and early fatigue means less energy.

There are some people who worry that they will get too little salt. But there is absolutely no cause for concern. Practically everything you eat contains some salt. The average American's largest supply of salt (other than that which he sprinkles on his food) comes from pork, ham, and bacon. One serving of ham provides you with as much as two grams of salt, so you can see that replacing salt naturally is not all that difficult. Most cheeses also have a high level of salt and are a good, natural way for replacing salt. Fruits generally do not have a high salt content, but the banana stands above all others as a good supply of salt. Most vegetables do not have a great deal of natural salt in them either, but endive greens, lettuce, potatoes, and spinach offer higher amounts of salt than other vegetables. In addition, there are many foods that are little else than carriers of salt. These include olives, pickles, relishes, luncheon meats, and dried beef. If you are concerned about not getting enough salt due to an excess of sweating and/or of high-humidity exercise, choosing foods from Table 12-1 will help replace that salt.

Table 12-1 illustrates that much of what you eat contains sodium. So salt replacement is not necessary. If you feel you need extra salt, get it from the natural, wholesome foods on the list, (marked by an asterisk), rather than by salting foods.

At one time salt tablets were recommended for people who sweated a great deal, but no more. The salt in salt tablets is too concentrated and causes problems. When exercising in a humid environment, more water is lost than salt. This causes an increase in salt concentration in the body. Additional salt will only widen the gap. So high salt intake is not necessary except for those who exercise in an extremely hot environment over a long period of time, and the use of salt tablets is not recommended at all. There are exceptions, but as a general rule you can assume that the less salt you eat, the better off you will be.

TABLE 12-1
High Salt Foods

All canned and frozen
  foods
Bacon
Beets*
Bouillon cubes
Canned meats
Canned soups or
  stews
Carrots*
Caviar
Celery salt
Cheese*
Chili sauce
Commercial salad
  dressings
Commercially made:
    Breads

Rolls
  Crackers
Dandelion greens*
Frankfurters and sausages
Garlic salt
Gravy
Ham
Kale*
Ketchup
Luncheon meats
Meat sauces
Milk*
Mustard
Mustard greens*
Olives
Onion salt
Organ meats

Pickled foods (sauerkraut)
Pickles
Pretzels
Relishes
Salt pork
Salted butter
Salted, dried, and smoked
  fish and meats
Salted nuts
Salted popcorn
Salted margarine
Shellfish
Soy sauce
Spinach*
Tenderizers
Worcestershire sauce

*Foods with naturally high content of salt.

Caffeine

Every morning, approximately 80 percent of America's adult population try to clear the cobwebs with that traditional "pick me up" cup of coffee. By noon, a good share of those 101 million people have had two to five cups of the warm beverage and, along with it, a liberal dose of caffeine. While there may be nothing better than the smell of coffee perking on the stove, drinking it can seriously affect your supply of energy.

Most people who drink coffee think it has a stimulating effect. The regular coffee drinker suggests he can't get started without his first cup in the morning. Indeed, initial research seems to support the claim that the caffeine in a cup of coffee produces a noticeable stimulus to the nervous system. Moreover, laboratory experiments indicate that coffee increases mental alertness, speeds reaction time, and actually helps people think more clearly. In short, caffeine has a stimulant effect on the brain and nervous system. Researchers are not sure exactly why this happens, but it may be that the caffeine in coffee increases the concentration of cyclic AMP. Cyclic AMP's role in the body is to stimulate cell activity, including the production of the hormones and the brain cells that play a role in alertness.

Along with these apparent benefits, caffeine may improve your performance in endurance events such as marathon running. It has been shown that caffeine promotes an increased release of fatty acids from the fatty tissues. That means that muscle glycogen will be spared, which will slow the onset of fatigue. Such information indicates a cup of coffee may be a great way to stay alert, run a better marathon, or provide you with energy.

Before jumping to conclusions, however, it is always best to consider the other side of the research. The culprit in coffee is caffeine, which is chemically known as 1, 3, 7-trimethylxanthine. Last year, Americans ingested 34 million pounds of this substance. When even small amounts of this substance enter your body, they begin to create some changes. After the initial perk to your cardiovascular system, caffeine goes to work on your muscles. They react to this new chemical by tensing up. In fact, even three to five hours after your last cup of coffee, your metabolism can remain increased from 10 to 25 percent. That means you are using more energy even though you may not be working any harder than normal. The cumulative effect contributes to that "tired, worn-out" feeling at the end of the day.

Still another energy-related problem is insomnia. The primary ingredient in over-the-counter "pep pills" is caffeine. College students quickly discover that a few cups of strong, black coffee will help them stay up all night to study for an exam. The student rationalizes this practice by saying he can get more sleep the next day. The executive, however, who drinks up to eight cups of coffee throughout the day and suffers with sleeplessness that night still has to get up for work the next day—feeling very tired. It's a pattern of living that's devastating to your energy supply: the coffee increases your metabolism, constantly picking you up throughout the day then dropping you in a tired heap throughout the evening, only to keep you up all night. Additionally, some scientists report that caffeine may influence certain brain receptors in such a way that they block the brain's own tranquilizing hormone. The result is increased anxiety.

Most people who drink coffee realize that it takes a lot more caffeine than is found in a cup or two of coffee to produce those results. The average cup of coffee contains only 100 to 150 mg. of caffeine, a relatively harmless amount. However, the average coffee drinker goes through two to three cups a day, pushing the amount of caffeine to 200 to 450 mg. Moreover, you may be getting caffeine from other sources such as tea, cola drinks, or cocoa. Compounding the problem is the fact that your body develops an immunity to those "good" boosts in alertness and reaction time. That is why the two to three-cup a day coffee drinker can easily increase his consumption to six to eight cups a day. And the dose of caffeine jumps close to the 1,000-mg. level that can produce dizziness, restlessness, irritability, and tremors.

Of course, different people handle caffeine in different ways. Some people seem to be able to drink large amounts of coffee and still don't experience skipped heart beats, anxiety, insomnia, and the jitters. There are other people who take one cup of coffee and are so hyped up that they swear off coffee for the rest of their lives.

There are several reasons for this. Some people can simply tolerate coffee better than others. It's that way with anything in life. And it's probably the same thing with caffeine. The difference is probably due to some obscure biochemical phenomenon of the individual. Then there are people who find that their brain is not nearly as sensitive to caffeine as others are. Again, this is probably due to some biochemical difference. And, like any other drug, people do develop a tolerance for caffeine. Consequently, they do not show the usual symptoms of caffeine stimulation. Yet, while their body may have adapted so that they're not aware of caffeine effects, their body may still be reacting in a harmful way that reduces their energy levels. If you drink coffee, recollect how many cups it used to take to stimulate you. If at one time one cup seemed to perk you up and now it takes two or more, you can conclude that your body is adapting to the amount of caffeine.

Does this mean you need to give up coffee entirely in your quest for more energy? Eventually, that might be a good goal. But a more sensible approach right now would be to try and cut back a little. If you are drinking ten cups of coffee a day, see if you can reduce that to five or six cups. At the same time, be more aware of the other sources of caffeine such as colas, tea, or cocoa. Once you notice the benefits of getting by with a little less caffeine, you will probably become more encouraged to cut back even a little more. If you can limit your daily intake of coffee to three cups or less, and make sure you aren't getting more from other sources, that amount of caffeine may not seriously affect your energy level.

Coffee is not the only caffeine culprit. As Table 12.2 indicates, a cup of tea contains between 60 to 75 mg. of caffeine depending upon whether you're using instant, leaf, or bag tea. Cocoa contains up to 50 mg. of caffeine and many cola drinks contain anywhere between 40 to 60 mg.

Americans consume excessive amounts of caffeine beginning at a very early age. Children eat or drink huge quantities of caffeine from soft drinks, candy bars, and colas. Thus a young child may weigh only 40 to 50 pounds and

TABLE 12-2
Common Sources of Caffeine*

	Milligrams
Beverage (Six-Ounce Cup)	
Brewed Coffee	100–150
Instant Coffee	86–89
Tea	60–75
Cola Drinks	40–60 per glass (8 oz.)
Decaffeinated Coffee	2–4
Over-The-Counter Analgesics	
Anacin, Aspirin, Bromo Seltzer	32 per tablet
Cope, Easy-Mens, Midol	32 per tablet
Vanquish	32 per tablet
Excedrin	60 per tablet
Pre-Mens	66 per tablet
Many Over-The-Counter Cold Remedies	30 per tablet
Many Over-The-Counter Stimulants	100 per tablet

*SOURCE: From *Executive Fitness*, 28 August 1979, Rodale Press.

very likely consume the caffeine equivalent for his body weight of an adult drinking eight cups of coffee each day. If your child is irritable, nervous, or doesn't sleep well, it's very likely that caffeine is the culprit. The excessive energy that you think your child has may really be symptomatic of too much caffeine. On the other hand, some research suggests that children may have an opposite response to caffeine—lethargy. Regardless, keep the caffeine content low with young children. Otherwise, it'll eventually wipe them out.

Dieting

The less said about dieting the better. Dieting is the pits when it comes to energy. Most dieters skip meals—breakfast in particular. Then they have a mid-morning snack or wait until noon to eat. This means that they probably have gone 15 hours or more without any food. No wonder that by 11:00 A.M. or so they feel famished, irritable—AND tired. Low blood sugar might be the cause, or it might just be the lack of carbohydrates. Unfortunately, at this time most people have a sweet roll and coffee. And they may put a little cream and some sugar in the coffee. The result is a temporary lift and then a big let down all because of the exhausting combination of fat, sugar, and caffeine, a deadly triad. To break this cycle, eat a decent breakfast or at coffee break time eat some fresh fruit, vegetables, or cheese.

Diets also tend to restrict the eating of certain foods—carbohydrates in particular. You need carbohydrates for energy levels. The cutting out of other foods may short-change you on vitamins and minerals.

Most dieters are tired all the time. The only thing that keeps them going and gives them a lift is when they see the weight drop on the scale and a change in the size of their clothing. Unfortunately, 90 to 95 percent of all diets fail. They do so because people cannot fight the overwhelming fatigue that's associated with dieting, and also the basic human drive for food.

Eating is OK—honest. Just don't skip meals and make sure that you eat the right balance of energy givers, and cut back on the energy robbers.

A Three Phase Plan for Eating for Energy

Many nutritionists base their recommendations for eating on the four basic food groups (milk, meat, bread-cereal, and vegetable-fruit), which were introduced in the mid 1950s in an effort to tranlate the many nutrient recommendations into simple food choices. In the Three Phase Eating For Energy Plan, those four basic food groups have been expanded to seven so that you will be certain to enjoy a complete and nutritious diet. While everyone likes a snack now and then, if you follow the eating chart you will reduce your intake of energy-robbing snacks.

Phase One is contained in the chart below. The left hand column notates a basic food group. Column 1 lists foods which may be eaten any time while foods in Column 2 should be consumed only in moderation.

Important Note: Whenever you are given a choice of several options and are allowed a certain amount weekly or monthly, make sure you follow the recommended number of servings. For example, under phase I Group 5, you are allowed a total of 2 to 3 servings of the various meats listed. That does not mean 2 to 3 servings of herring, 2 to 3 servings of mackerel, 2 to 3 servings of salmon, etc. If you have one serving of herring, one serving of mackerel, and one serving of salmon throughout the week, that is your limit for that week. The same holds true for all options throughout each phase.

Phase One

		Anytime	2–3 Times a Week
1 or more servings a day	Group 1 **Dark green, leafy, and yellow vegetables.** Such as asparagus, broccoli, carrots, chicory, collards, green peas, kale, mustard greens, parsley, pumpkins, rutabagas, spinach, squash, string beans, sweet potatoes, and wax beans.	All fresh and frozen vegetables such as those listed on the left.	Salted vegetable juices, i.e., V-8 juice, or salted canned soups and vegetables. May have 2–3 servings a week total.

Plan for Eating for Energy—Continued

Phase One—Continued

		Anytime	2–3 Times a Week
1 or more servings a day	**Group 2** **Citrus fruits, raw cabbage, and salad greens.** Such as berries, cabbage, cantaloupe, celery, grapefruit, green peppers, lemons, lettuce, limes, mangoes, oranges, papayas, and tomatoes.	All frozen and fresh citrus fruits, cabbage, and salad greens. Juices are also permitted.	Salted tomato juice, sweetened berry, lemon, grapefruit, orange, etc., juices.
1 or more servings a day	**Group 3a** **Potatoes and other vegetables not listed in Groups 1 and 2.** Such as beets, corn, cucumbers, eggplant, onions, parsnips, potatoes, and white turnips.	All fresh and frozen vegetables such as those listed on the left.	Sweetened and salted canned vegetables.
1 or more servings a day	**Group 3b** **Noncitrus fruits.** Such as apples, bananas, figs, grapes, peaches, pears, pineapples, plums, prunes, and raisins. Juices are permitted.	All fresh and frozen fruits such as those listed on the left.	Avocado, fruits canned in syrup, sweetened fruits and juices.

Plan for Eating for Energy—Continued

Phase One—Continued

		Anytime	2–3 Times a Week
2 or more servings a day	Group 4 **Milk and milk products.**	Buttermilk, farmer or pot cheese, low-fat cottage cheese, low-fat milk with 1% milk fat, skim milk, and ricotta skim milk.	Frozen low-fat yogurt, low-fat milk with 2% milk fat, low-fat (2%) yogurt plain or sweetened, and regular cottage cheese (4% milk fat). Hard cheeses: blue, brick, camembert, cheddar (note: part-skim mozzarella and part-skim ricotta are preferable but still rich in fat), ice cream, ice milk, processed cheese, whole milk, and whole milk yogurt.
2 servings (about 4 oz. total) a day	Group 5 **Meats, poultry, fish, dried beans, rice, lentils, soybeans, peas, nuts, peanut butter, and eggs.**	Chicken or turkey (no skin). Fish such as cod, flounder, haddock, halibut, perch, pollock, rockfish, shellfish (except shrimp), sole, tuna (water-packed), egg whites, rice, and lentils.	Fish such as herring, mackerel, salmon, sardines, shrimp, and tuna (oil-packed). Red meat such as flank steak, ham, leg of lamb, plate beef, round steak, rump roast, sirloin steak, veal, soybeans, and peanut butter. Deep-fried and breaded fish and poultry, bacon, corned beef, ground beef, hot dogs, liver, liverwurst, pork loin, salami, sausage, spareribs, untrimmed meats, luncheon meats, egg yolks, or whole eggs.

Plan for Eating for Energy—Continued

Phase One—Continued

		Anytime	2–3 Times a Week
2 or more servings a day	Group 6 **Whole grain breads and cereals.**	Barley, bread and rolls (whole grain), bulghur, oatmeal, pasta, whole grain cereal (except granola).	Granola cereals, white breads, and traditional packaged cereals.
2 to 4 servings a day	Group 7 **Vegetable oils and fats.**	Margarines made with nonhydrogenated soybean oil.	Mayonnaise, salad oils, and soft tub margarines. Butter, cream, cream cheese, lard, and sour cream.
	Snack Foods	. . .	Angel food cake, animal crackers, fig bars, gingerbread, gingersnaps, popcorn (with small amounts of salt and butter), and sherbet. Chocolate, coconut, commercial pies, pastries, donuts, potato chips, and soda pop.

Phase Two is similar to Phase One. The difference is that some less energetic foods have been shifted to the right, out of the "anytime" and "moderation" columns. These are foods that you may have been reluctant to give up at first, but as you added more nutritious energy givers to your diet, you found that you have replaced some of the poor-quality foods you once ate.

Plan for Eating for Energy—Continued
Phase Two

		Anytime	2–3 Times a Week	Once a Week
1 or more servings a day	**Group 1** **Dark green, leafy, and yellow vegetables.** Such as asparagus, broccoli, carrots, chicory, collards, green peas, kale, mustard greens, parsley, pumpkins, rutabagas, spinach, squash, string beans, sweet potatoes, and wax beans.	All fresh and frozen vegetables such as those listed on the left.	Salted vegetable juices, i.e., V-8 juice, or salted canned soups and vegetables. May have 2–3 servings a week total.	. . .
1 or more servings a day	**Group 2** **Citrus fruits, raw cabbage, and salad greens.** Such as berries, cabbage, cantaloupe, celery, grapefruit, green peppers, lemons, lettuce, limes, mangoes, oranges, papayas, and tomatoes.	All frozen and fresh citrus fruits, cabbage, and salad greens. Juices are also permitted.	Salted tomato juice, sweetened berry, lemon, grapefruit, orange, etc., juices.	. . .

Plan for Eating for Energy—Continued

Phase Two—Continued

		Anytime	2–3 Times a Week	Once a Week
1 or more servings a day	Group 3a **Potatoes and other vegetables not listed in Groups 1 and 2.** Such as beets, corn, cucumbers, eggplant, onions, parsnips, potatoes, and white turnips.	All fresh and frozen vegetables such as those listed on the left.	Sweetened and salted canned vegetables.	French fries, olives, and pickles.
1 or more servings a day	Group 3b **Noncitrus fruits.** Such as apples, bananas, figs, grapes, peaches, pears, pineapples, plums, prunes, and raisins. Juices are permitted.	All fresh and frozen fruits such as those listed on the left.	Avocado, fruits canned in syrup, sweetened fruits and juices.	. . .

Plan for Eating for Energy—Continued

Phase Two—Continued

		Anytime	2–3 Times a Week	Once a Week
2 or more servings a day	Group 4 **Milk and milk products.**	Buttermilk, farmer or pot cheese, low-fat cottage cheese, low-fat milk with 1% milk fat, skim milk, and ricotta skim milk.	Frozen low-fat yogurt, low-fat milk with 2% milk fat, low-fat (2%) yogurt plain or sweetened, and regular cottage cheese (4% milk fat).	Hard cheeses: blue, brick, camembert, cheddar (note: part-skim mozzarella and part-skim ricotta are preferable but still rich in fat), ice cream, ice milk, processed cheese, whole milk, and whole milk yogurt.
2 servings (about 4 oz. total) a day	Group 5 **Meats, poultry, fish, dried beans, rice, lentils, soybeans, peas, nuts, peanut butter, and eggs.**	Chicken or turkey (no skin). Fish such as cod, flounder, haddock, halibut, perch, pollock, rockfish, shellfish (except shrimp), sole, tuna (water-packed), egg whites, rice, and lentils.	Fish such as herring, mackerel, salmon, sardines, shrimp, and tuna (oil-packed). Red meat such as flank steak, ham, leg of lamb, plate beef, round steak, rump roast, sirloin steak, veal, soybeans, and peanut butter.	Deep-fried and breaded fish and poultry, bacon, corned beef, ground beef, hot dogs, liver, liverwurst, pork loin, salami, sausage, spareribs, untrimmed meats, luncheon meats, egg yolks, or whole eggs.

Plan for Eating for Energy—Continued

Phase Two—Continued

		Anytime	2–3 Times a Week	Once a Week
2 or more servings a day	**Group 6 Whole grain breads and cereals.**	Barley, bread and rolls (whole grain), bulghur, oatmeal, pasta, whole grain cereal (except granola).	Granola cereals.	White breads, and traditional packaged cereals.
2 to 4 servings a day	**Group 7 Vegetable oils and fats.**	Margarines made with nonhydrogenated soybean oil.	Mayonnaise, salad oils, and soft tub margarines.	Butter, cream, cream cheese, lard, and sour cream.
	Snack Foods	. . .	Angel food cake, animal crackers, fig bars, gingerbread, gingersnaps, popcorn (with small amounts of salt and butter), and sherbet.	Chocolate, coconut, commercial pies, pastries, donuts, potato chips, and soda pop.

Phase Three is the *Maximum Personal Energy* diet. It is low in processed and refined foods and high in fresh and frozen fruits and vegetables. It is high in complex carbohydrates and low in fat. In this phase, virtually all sugar and salt have been eliminated from your regular eating pattern, though now and then you may feel free to dip into your passion food barrel you once subsisted on.

Plan for Eating for Energy—Continued
Phase Three

		Anytime	2–3 Times a Week	Once a Week	Once a Month
1 or more servings a day	Group 1 **Dark green, leafy, and yellow vegetables.** Such as asparagus, broccoli, carrots, chicory, collards, green peas, kale, mustard greens, parsley, pumpkins, rutabagas, spinach, squash, string beans, sweet potatoes, and wax beans.	All fresh and frozen vegetables such as those listed on the left.	Salted vegetable juices, i.e., V-8 juice, salted canned soups and vegetables.	Salted vegetable juices, i.e., V-8 juice, or salted canned soups and vegetables. May have 2–3 servings a week total.	. . .
1 or more servings a day	Group 2 **Citrus fruits, raw cabbage, and salad greens.** Such as berries, cabbage, cantaloupe, celery, grapefruit, green peppers, lemons, lettuce, limes, mangoes, oranges, papayas, and tomatoes.	All frozen and fresh citrus fruits, cabbage, and salad greens. Juices are also permitted.	Sweetened berry, lemon, grapefruit, orange, etc., juices.	Salted tomato juice.	. . .

Plan for Eating for Energy—Continued

Phase Three—Continued

		Anytime	2–3 Times a Week	Once a Week	Once a Month
1 or more servings a day	Group 3a **Potatoes and other vegetables not listed in Groups 1 and 2.** Such as beets, corn, cucumbers, eggplant, onions, parsnips, potatoes, and white turnips.	All fresh and frozen vegetables such as those listed on the left.	Sweetened and canned vegetables.	Salted canned vegetables.	French fries, olives, and pickles.
1 or more servings a day	Group 3b **Noncitrus fruits.** Such as apples, bananas, figs, grapes, peaches, pears, pineapples, plums, prunes, and raisins. Juices are permitted.	All fresh and frozen fruits such as those listed on the left.	Sweetened fruit juice.	Avocados, fruits canned in syrup, and sweetened fruit.	. . .

Plan for Eating for Energy—Continued

Phase Three—Continued

		Anytime	2–3 Times a Week	Once a Week	Once a Month
2 or more servings a day	Group 4 Milk and milk products.	Buttermilk, farmer or pot cheese, low-fat cottage cheese, low-fat milk with 1% milk fat, skim milk, and ricotta skim milk.	Frozen low-fat yogurt, low-fat milk with 2% milk fat, low-fat (2%) yogurt plain or sweetened, and regular cottage cheese (4% milk fat).	Hard cheeses: blue, brick, camembert, cheddar (note: part-skim mozzarella and part-skim ricotta are preferable but still rich in fat), ice milk, processed cheese, whole milk, and whole milk yogurt.	Ice cream
2 servings (about 4 oz. total) a day	Group 5 Meats, poultry, fish, dried beans, rice, lentils, soybeans, peas, nuts, peanut butter, and eggs.	Chicken or turkey (no skin). Fish such as cod, flounder, haddock, halibut, perch, pollock, rockfish, shellfish (except shrimp), sole, tuna (water-packed), egg whites, rice, and lentils.	Fish such as herring, mackerel, salmon, sardines, shrimp, and tuna (oil-packed). Red meat such as flank steak, ham, leg of lamb, plate beef, round steak, rump roast, sirloin steak, veal, soybeans, and peanut butter.	Deep-fried and breaded fish and poultry, ground beef, liver, pork loin, spareribs, untrimmed meats, egg yolks or whole eggs.	Bacon, corned beef, hot dogs, salami, sausage, luncheon meats, i.e., bologna, and liverwurst.

Plan for Eating for Energy—Continued

Phase Three—Continued

		Anytime	2–3 Times a Week	Once a Week	Once a Month
2 or more servings a day	Group 6 **Whole grain breads and cereals.**	Barley, bread and rolls (whole grain), bulghur, oatmeal, pasta, whole grain cereal (except granola).	Unsweetened granola cereals.	Sweetened granola and traditional packaged cereals.	Pre-sweet-ened cereals and white bread.
2 to 4 servings a day	Group 7 **Vegetable oils and fats.**	Margarines made with nonhydroge-nated soybean oil.	Mayonnaise, salad oils, and soft tub margarines.	Butter, cream, cream cheese, and sour cream.	Lard.
	Snack Foods	. . .	. . .	Angel food cake, animal crackers, fig bars, gingerbread, gingersnaps, popcorn (with small amounts of salt and butter), and sherbet.	Choco-late, co-conut, com-mercial pies, pastries, donuts, potato chips, and soda pop.

Note: A nutrition purist might criticize our inclusion of selected foods 1–3 times per week (foods that contain sugar, salt, and saturated fats). This plan, however, takes into consideration that maintaining a prudent, energy-giving diet is sometimes difficult in our society. It is designed to help a person select the best possible foods from a variety of choices. Also, you must remember that few foods are entirely good or bad. Milk is a nutritious beverage, yet contains high levels of saturated fats. Rather than cut milk out of your diet entirely, this plan recommends a limit to the amount of whole milk you drink. At Phase II, the plan meets the U.S. Senate nutrition guidelines and at Phase III it exceeds them.

SLIMMING FOR ENERGY

CHAPTER 13
Fat and Where It's At

If you'd look around and start identifying people who seem to be dynamos of energy, you would notice one thing: Most are slim and trim, no protruding stomachs, no "orange peel" skin, no flabby arms and spongy thighs. That in itself should tell you something about the relationship between energy and obesity. People who have an overabundance of body fat generally do not have the energy of one who has only a small percentage of body fat.

Fat, as you learned in Chapter 11, is important and functional. It acts as your energy storehouse. This stored fat gives you energy for the long run—or for chopping wood, walking long distances, playing tennis for several hours, or digging a ditch all day long. That is the good news of fat. The bad news is that too much fat can rob you of energy. Here's how.

Fat as an Energy Robber

The fat cells of your body are your fuel storage tanks. When you burn off fewer calories through activity than your body takes in, you convert these extra calories into fat. This fat then gets deposited in your fat cells. To illustrate this point, suppose that you eat 2,400 calories worth of food during a 24-hour period, and your level of activity is such that you burn off exactly 2,400 calories as you work, sleep, and play your way through the day. Supply and demand are equal. Your body neither calls on reserves to make up an energy deficit, nor does it deposit extra calories in the form of fat. You are maintaining your weight. However, if you consume 2,400 calories and burn off only 2,300 of them, your body will convert those 100 unnecessary calories of food into fat and "store" it until such time as it is needed for energy.

One pound of fat is the equivalent of 3,500 unnecessary calories. Whether these calories are eaten in the form of sirloin steak, ice cream, or raw carrots makes no difference. A calorie is a calorie. With this in mind, you can see that if you eat 100 calories a day more than you burn off through physical activity, at the end of 35 days, you'll have gained a pound. If you continue at the same rate, you'll be ten pounds heavier at the end of the year.

Fat is okay, provided it does not exceed 15 percent (men) or 19 percent (women) of your overall weight. When it exceeds that range it puts a drain on your energy levels—not before.

When excess fat is put on, there is more body tissue to take care of. Your various body systems, that is, muscles, bones, heart, and lungs, are under a strain to support the additional load. Think of it: If you had to carry an extra 20- to 30-pound pack on your back each day, your body would soon rebel. Well it's no different with fat. Excess fat is considered a "pack on the back." Your skeletal and muscle systems are under strain to support the additional load. Your heart and lungs must work harder in order to assist your muscles in moving all the fat around. For example the extra fat causes your resting and working heart rate to be higher. For many people it may be 10 to 30 beats higher for any task. Anything from sweeping the floors to climbing stairs. That means your heart may beat 14,000 to 42,000 times more per day. Even your breathing rate increases. Scientists tell us that a person who carries too much fat will probably take 2 to 3 more breaths per minute, even when sleeping. This is 2,800 to 4,400 more breaths per day.

It's the same way with your muscles and bones. Think about the last time you backpacked, climbed a mountain, or carried a suitcase through an airport terminal. After a short time you wanted to rest. The first thing you did was take the pack off your back or put the suitcase down. Why? Your muscles ached. They were screaming for rest and more oxygen.

The extra fat problem, unfortunately, goes beyond extra breaths, heart beats, and tired muscles and bones. Excess fat can cause problems to the arteries themselves. The build up of fat in the vessels is an energy-robbing by-product of being fat. While fat is constantly transported throughout your blood vessels to be deposited in the fat cells of your body, too much fat heightens the possibility that the walls of your arteries will accumulate the fat, thus restricting the blood flow in the artery. It's much like an old pipe which is starting to clog up with rust and mineral deposits.

The clogging of the arteries slows the blood supply to the muscles, organs, and other tissues. As a result the body becomes less efficient. The clogging also causes the blood vessels to lose their elasticity or flexibility. The walls tear and thicken with plaques so that the vessels are narrowed even more. The blood must be pushed with greater force to continue circulation. This condition is called peripheral resistance. The heart is forced to work harder. Blood pressure increases. Sometimes small vessels are entirely blocked, and circulation to these peripheral areas of the body is cut off. Thus the poor circulation and "cold feet" of some people may occur. But the feet and hands are not the only places where these vessels are located. They are also found in the heart, the brain, and in various other organs. The result is less efficiency and more fatigue.

As the fatty deposits continue to progress and the loss of flexibility becomes more significant, the circulatory system gets even more sluggish. Heart rate and blood pressure start to rise. The blood vessels become less elastic and breathing becomes more shallow. In short, cardiovascular fitness drops and early fatigue sets in. Physical effort becomes a chore, even if it is done lying down. Many times, extra effort coupled with an emotionally charged situation causes a very high heart rate and blood pressure. People feel uncomfortable—dizzy or "shaky." Many may be frightened by this feeling. Consequently, less physical work is done. With less exercise there is a further decrease in cardiovascular fitness. A vicious cycle ensues: less work, less fitness, more fatigue, less work. Soon people become so unfit that they avoid exercise at all costs. They simply don't have the stamina to keep it up any longer.

Research suggests that obese people have higher levels of insulin circulating in their blood than do nonobese people. Significantly, however, the obese person also secretes more insulin after eating. This phenomenon of more insulin in the blood and being released is important. Insulin not only removes extra glucose from the bloodstream, it also makes you feel sleepy and downtrodden. You have less energy.

A quick review shows there are many physiological energy-draining syndromes that result from being too fat:

1. Muscles and bones must labor under great strain.
2. Heart and lungs must work harder to assist muscles.
3. Blood pressure increases, causing physical fatigue.
4. Blood vessels become less elastic, further decreasing circulation.
5. Fatty deposits build up on blood vessel linings.
6. Extra fat can cause problems with insulin.

But fatness goes beyond these physical reasons as an energy drain. Fatness causes emotional fatigue. Self-concepts and relationships have been destroyed by unwanted bulges and bumps. It seems the fatter people get, the sadder they get.

Fat and Emotional Fatigue

Poor self-concepts and lousy interpersonal relationships can lead to the blues. The blues are soon followed by despondency, depression, and ultimately, fatigue. Psychologists tell us that self-esteem is important in determining your overall energy levels. In our society, being told you have an expanding waistline, wide hips, or unattractive thighs is the equivalent of being insulted. You resent it. You hate it. You end up despising your body, yourself, and the world.

The stress brought on by this attitude is vicious. Stress, or depression, causes overeating in those people who have learned to eat under stressful conditions. Many times they are called binge eaters. The overeating causes them to consume more calories than they burn off. An increase in fatness ensues. With an increase in fatness people become less active, which results in no natural outlet for their stress. Thereby, a *Catch-22* syndrome is completed.

Additionally, those who carry too much body fat are often tagged with the incorrect term "lazy." They're far from lazy. These poor, tired individuals are struggling through life with a distinct, energy-robbing burden. They're not lazy, just overloaded psychologically and physically, and consequently they're worn out.

Fat and Weight

You may have noticed that I never mention being overweight. Instead, I refer to a condition of obesity, or too much body fat. This is an important distinction, and one you need to understand to discuss the concept of slimming

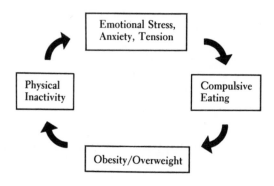

to increase energy. Let me begin by tossing two apparently contradictory statements at you:

A person can be underweight, yet obese.

A person can be overweight and not obese.

Sounds confusing, doesn't it? That's because for so long we have been slaves to the scales and the height/weight charts so that we have failed to understand the concept of lean body tissue. What we should be concerned about is fat, not weight.

Being overweight is merely weighing more than the standardized height/weight tables put out by insurance companies that tell you what you should weigh. Being obese refers to the percentage of fat that is on your body. There is a big difference. For example, you can have two men who are 6'2" tall and weigh 235 pounds. One man plays halfback for the Los Angeles Rams and the other is a less active male citizen. According to the height/weight charts, both are overweight since they shouldn't exceed 198 pounds. However, when you ask both men to take off their shirts, there is an obvious difference between the two. The professional football player has minimal body fat and a high distribution of lean body tissue. He looks very good. The other gentleman carries a large amount of fat and has very little lean body tissue. He doesn't look so good. Yet according to the charts, both are in the same "shape."

Women usually face this problem in reverse. They panic at the sight of an unwanted pound. Yet in their fight to ward off pounds, they've ignored what happens to their bodies. Consequently, they may stay at a respectable 115 pounds but move up another dress size. In other words, they're adept at losing weight but not fat. They have lost lean body tissue yet gained body fat.

The key, you see, is lean body tissue, the bone, organ, and muscle tissue of your body. While you can't do much about your bones and organs, you can control the amount of muscle tissue you have. A person in good physical condition will have a high distribution of lean body tissue and a low distribution of fat. A person who is unfit will have a reverse distribution.

Now that puts a different twist in the whole weight-loss issue. For you see, you need to lose fat, not weight. Unfortunately, you cannot assume that losing weight automatically means that you're losing fat. What you can assume, however, is that when you lose weight through dieting you will lose both fat and lean body tissue. Hence, you become a scaled down version of the original model: 30 pounds lighter but still plagued with sagging muscles, a protruding stomach, flabby thighs, and a lack of energy.

Drs. Bill Zuti and Lawrence Golding, conducted a study at Kent State University that illustrates this point nicely. The research team set out to compare the effects of several different methods of weight reduction on body weight, body composition, and selected blood measurements. The 25 women participating in the study were all between the ages of 25 and 40, and were 20 to 40 pounds overfat. Three groups were formed: 1) eight women were put on a diet to reduce their caloric intake by 500 calories per day, but they held their physical activity constant; 2) nine continued to eat as usual, but increased their physical activity to burn off 500 extra calories a day; and 3) eight reduced caloric intake by 250 calories a day and increased their physical activity to burn off 250 calories a day. Before and after the 16-week period, the subjects were tested for body weight, body density, skinfold and girth measurements, and selected blood fats.

The results indicated that there were no significant differences between the groups in the amount of weight lost. In all three groups the average individual loss was 11.4 pounds. Thus, the study indicated that all of the methods were extremely effective in controlling weight. However, the significant finding of the study was that there was a difference between the groups with regard to body composition. Those in the exercise group and in the combination exercise/diet group had undergone significant changes in body density. The dieting group lost both body fat and muscle tissue; the exercise group lost more body fat and no muscle tissue. The report concluded that the use of exercise in a weight reduction program is far superior to dieting alone in its effect on body composition.

When people lose weight by dieting they often remain flabby. But if you exercise while you diet or use exercise as the means for losing weight, your muscles will be much firmer. Therefore, you will look and feel better after losing weight through exercise than you will after just dieting.

The reason for this lies in an understanding of the fat-loss principle. Basically, there is one way to lose fat: establish a caloric deficit. That simply means that you burn off more calories than you eat. Of course, no one "eats" a calorie. We eat potatoes, meat, pies, and the rest, which require the use of a certain amount of energy. If the calories in these foods are not used, they are stored as fat. To lose the extra poundage, you have two choices: decrease the amount of food you eat, or increase the amount of calories you use.

The Woes of Dieting

The most obvious and most often used method to lose extra poundage is to diet. It seems to make sense. "If I'm 500 calories over my limit, the best way to lose weight is to cut 500 calories out of my daily diet. Cut back on portions, no desserts, and no snacks." The only problem is that 95 percent of those people who lose weight through dieting gain it right back. The reasons why follow.

First, dieting is "unnatural." It works against the body's own wants and needs. You are a creature that is made to eat. Eventually your body will cry for more food and you will respond. Hence, the diet is disregarded. In addition to being unnatural, dieting is loaded with psychological stumbling blocks. Eating has been linked to emotional needs that are as compelling as actual hunger. We eat when we're nervous. We eat when we're bored. We reward ourselves with food when we are happy. We soothe ourselves with a big meal when we are sad. As children, we were good little boys or girls if we cleaned up our plates. We could have a candy bar if we behaved. Our Little League coaches even took us to the ice cream stand if we won the ball game. So the very act of dieting is psychologically interpreted as punishment, and no one likes to be punished for very long.

In addition to all that, dieting simply goes against everything our culture demands from us. In our society, food is plentiful. It's everywhere. It's also big business. "You're the one," because "you deserve a break today," so why not have a hamburger, a malted shake, or french fries? Radio, TV, magazine advertisements, and giant billboards all proclaim food as being fun and readily available right around the corner. Food advertisers know how to appeal to our cravings in a way that only the strongest can resist.

There's one other reason I'm down on diets, and that is that dieting robs you of energy. You see, we have been so conditioned about weight loss through dieting that we have forgotten the purpose of food. Simply stated, we *need* food to live, and we need a balanced, adequate amount of food each day in order to have the energy to carry out our daily activities. When a person who normally consumes 2,500 calories decides to starve off 250 of those calories each day, he is simply depriving himself of the fuel he needs to work and play. There is a good deal of indirect evidence to support this. If you'd take a look at the caloric requirement tables issued by the World Health Organization of the United Nations, you would see that they suggest 2,400 calories for a "sedentary" man while 4,500 calories are recommended for a "very active" man. Hard-working laborers, soldiers, and athletes require 6,000 or more calories per day, according to this organization. In other words, more "fuel" is needed for people who require a lot of energy. It has been estimated that Olympic-class swimmers must take in approximately 6,000 to 8,000 calories while on their grueling training. They require so much energy that without the extra fuel they would not be able to work as hard.

The implications are obvious. Dieting depletes our fuel supply, hence, creates an energy shortage. That shortage is experienced far too often by dieters and the result is a drastic reduction in activity and the drive to conserve fuel. It's like starting off in third gear. The engine barely has enough energy to get you going. I'm afraid that's the way many dieters feel.

Finally, dieting does not allow your body to look good. So you're still depressed, despondent, dejected, and de-energized. You may temporarily drop 15 or 20 pounds, but your body will still have that "soft" look. You may still have a bit of a midriff bulge or flabby thighs. That's because dieting does not discriminate. It takes off pounds whether they be muscle or fat. I'm sure you've heard some say, "I lose weight, but I lose it in all the wrong places." For women, this usually means the diet unloaded 4 pounds *and* two inches from her bust. For men, the bay window stayed while the biceps dwindled, adding to that pear-shaped, somewhat limpid look. The Golding-Zuti study I mentioned earlier illustrated just this point.

With all this going against you, why diet? I can see no sound reason to subject yourself to such energy-draining abuse, especially since there is an alternative, one that not only works directly to increase your energy, but is fun too! Instead of thinking negatively (don't eat this, none of that) think positively (add ten minutes here, treat yourself to an extra game of tennis). The key to slimming for energy is a regular program of aerobic activity.

Assessing Your Condition

Before beginning your program, you need to assess your condition. Are you indeed obese? There are a number of ways to find this out, but remember, we are concerned with fat, not body weight. Physiologists measure this in terms of percentages. As I mentioned before, ideally, a woman should have about 19 percent fat on her body, while a man should have 15 percent. If you exceed those percentages, you are accumulating too much fat. If a man exceeds 25 percent and a woman 29 percent, they enter the range of obesity, and a world of very little energy.

Measuring Skinfold Thickness

The National Center of Health Statistics in Washington points out that "skin folds permit a closer estimate of body fat than do the tables of relative weight. . . . Skin folds are becoming established as the easiest and most direct measure of body fat available in the doctor's office, the clinic, or in a large-scale population survey."

In most people under the age of 50, at least half of the body fat is stored directly underneath the skin. By measuring the thickness of the fold produced when the skin and tissue just under it are firmly grasped, it is possible to get a good idea of how much fat is present. Some of the most common locations at which this measurement is taken include the upper arm at the triceps (back of upper arm), the subscapular region (middle of the back at the shoulder blades), the waistline, the biceps (front of upper arm), and the ilium (waistline right above the hipbone).

The Pinch Test

Calipers are precise and scientific, but you're not conducting a research survey. You don't need a caliper to measure your own skinfold to determine whether or not you are fat. Simply do the pinch test.

Gently pinch the skin at the triceps of one upper arm (at the back), midway between the shoulder and elbow (with the thumb and forefinger of the other hand). Ideally, the skinfold should be between ¼ and ½ of an inch. If you can grasp more than 1 inch, you can probably conclude you are sliding into the obese range.

The Chest/Waist Test

Here's another way to tell if you're too fat. Stand with your shoulders pulled back and *maximum* chest expansion. Measure the circumference of your chest just below the armpits. Be certain your tape measure is flat and level. Then measure your waist (at the navel), with your stomach in a relaxed position —not sucked in or forced out. For men, the chest should be five inches greater in circumference than the waist; for women, the difference should be ten inches. If your chest/waist difference is *less* than the five or ten inch criteria, you can conclude that you are carrying too much fat.

Weight Gain Test

A third test is to simply recall what you weighed when you were 18 if you are a woman, or 21 if you are a man. If memory fails, you can dig out old medical records. You can assume that each pound gained since that time represents an accumulation of fat.

Note: If you were obese at 18 or 21 and have lost weight, this test doesn't apply. Furthermore, if you have gained a lot of weight because you have been on a weight-training program, the test will also be invalid.

The Mirror Test

The quickest, easiest way to find out if you are too fat is to get undressed and stand in front of a full length mirror. Be critical. Do you like what you see?

Have your body contours changed? If you look fat, you can reasonably conclude that you *are* fat. If you sag where you don't want to sag, if your abdomen protrudes, you're probably moving into the obese range or are already there. Ask yourself the following questions.

1. Does your stomach protrude?   Yes____ No____
2. Are your hips too big?   Yes____ No____
3. Do you have saddlebags on the tops of your thighs?   Yes____ No____
4. Do your breast or chest muscles sag?   Yes____ No____
5. Do you have handlebars above your hips?   Yes____ No____
6. Do the back of your arms seem flabby?   Yes____ No____
7. Do your legs seem to have the cottage cheese look?   Yes____ No____
8. Are your ankles too big?   Yes____ No____

If the answer is yes to any of these questions, you are probably carrying too much fat. Just be careful that you aren't too hard on yourself when you do the mirror test. Younger women especially are apt to want to measure up to a fashion model's ideal figure which, unless you are built along lean, long ectomorphic lines, is probably not possible nor even desirable.

The Jiggle Test

If the mirror test doesn't tell you too much, you might try running in place while standing in front of the mirror without your clothes on. Make sure no one's looking. If parts of your body jiggle and they're not supposed to, you can conclude that what you see jiggling is fat, and should be lost. If you still can't figure it out, look at your thighs, abdomen, and jowls or chin.

By now you should have a pretty good idea of whether or not you are carrying around too much fat to have the energy you would like to have. The problem, of course, is how to remove that fat so that you can really *live* rather than exist. Since my plan is based on *using* calories rather than restricting calories, activity is the foundation for getting rid of that energy-robbing fat. I'd like to tell you that it's easy, and that it's effortless. That's what all the advertisements say about the gadgets and pills that promise to melt away your fat. I have to be more realistic, though, and tell you that while using activity to reduce fat is easier than dieting, it still takes a degree of self-discipline and determination.

The Inches-Off, No-Diet Plan

Calories are quite familiar to people concerned about their weight. Most know which foods are low in calories and which foods have high caloric content. Many have memorized the exact caloric values of a wide variety of foods. In other words, the calorie has been thought of mainly as something one eats, but hardly ever as a unit of energy, as fuel to thrive on.

Although many people count the number of calories they eat each day, the idea of counting the number of calories they burn is relatively new. My entire fat-loss principle is predicated on burning more calories than you eat. The program depends on getting an initial bead on your individual caloric income and caloric outgo. While it would be ludicrous to claim that keeping track of the calories that one burns is fun, it is certainly no more difficult than the traditional routine of counting the number of calories consumed. It's just different.

Everything You Need to Know about Calories

The calories your body requires just to keep going may be quite a few more or less than what some other person's body needs to keep from grinding to a halt. One reason for this difference is your individual basal metabolic rate. Roughly defined, the basal metabolic rate is the rate of energy turnover— measured while the person is sleeping or at rest—necessary to sustain all of the body's vital processes. This basal metabolic rate, in turn, depends upon several factors. One of the most important factors is your body size. Most people who weigh from 100 to 120 pounds burn about 50 to 60 calories per hour while at rest. People who weigh from 150 to 170 pounds usually burn 65 to 80 calories per hour while at rest.

In the same way, one individual can burn a significantly different number of calories during activity than another person burns. Variations depend upon age, level of fitness, sex, skill, nutrition, environmental conditions and, very importantly, body size. For instance, during an hour of gardening, a 200-pounder will burn approximately 430 calories, while a person weighing 100 pounds will burn only about 285 calories—much the same as a large automobile uses more gas than a little economy model does to go the same distance.

How to Determine Your Caloric Outgo and Intake

The six Activity Tables in Appendix A entitled "The Fat-Loss Calorie Counter" take into account these individual differences. Start by looking at the column headed by the number of pounds you weigh. In that particular column are listed the number of calories you burn while participating in the various activities listed at the left side of the table. You can then use Appendix B, the Calorie Content of Food, to assess the number of calories you consume in your daily meals and snacks. By comparing the two figures, you'll get an idea of just how many net calories your body is exchanging and, perhaps, keeping as glycogen, or fat.

A local schoolteacher I know is a good example of this. (See Table 13-1.) In the warmer months, Ed is physically active on a regular basis. He does some running and cycling. He's more apt to walk rather than use his car. He plays tennis. On top of that, he enjoys working in his garden. Consequently, he has little trouble with excess fat. His eating habits don't change. In fact, it's not unusual for Ed to eat more during the summer than the winter. Yet the amount of calories he eats are balanced with the amount of calories he uses.

When winter rolls around, Ed becomes somewhat less active, nothing drastic. His bicycle stays in the garage. He finds the Michigan winter weather a bit too severe for running or walking outdoors. Of course, there's no garden work. He enjoys playing in a basketball league, but that's only once a week. Even though his eating habits remain the same, he always puts on a few unwanted pounds during the winter. That's because his caloric output has declined. He is not using as many calories as he does during the summer and he ends up with a surplus at the end of each day, only about 200 extra, in fact. But that's about two pounds of fat gained each month. A five-month winter could mean ten extra pounds for Ed.

To estimate your caloric expenditure, check Appendix A on page 274 to find out the number of calories you would burn if you slept 24 hours. This would be your basal caloric need. Add to this basal caloric need the following percentages, depending upon your personal lifestyle.

1. Add 20 percent to the basal caloric need for bed patients or people confined to wheelchairs.
2. Add 30 percent for individuals who have only limited physical exercise. These would include ambulatory hospital patients and people convalescing from serious illness.
3. Add 40 percent for individuals who are not convalescing, but are doing very little work. Most housewives who engage in many social activities and have someone to do their housework would fall into this category. Students and secretaries who do not engage in regular exercise would also fall into this category; most office workers who do not engage in

TABLE 13-1
Ed's Daily Caloric Exchange

Ed's Daily Intake

Breakfast	Calories
1 bowl cereal with milk and sugar	250
½ grapefruit	50
2 pieces of toast with butter and jam	280
2 cups of coffee with cream and sugar	96
Mid-morning Snack	
donut	150
2 cups of coffee with cream and sugar	96
Lunch	
2 sandwiches (cheese, tuna, etc.)	560
apple	75
2 cookies	65
After School	
1 cola	150
chips or peanuts	100
Supper	
salad with dressing	150
meat	200
rice or potato	100
glass of milk	250
dessert	200
Late Night Snack	
2 beers	300
nuts	50
TOTAL	**3,122**

Ed's Daily Output

Driving car	100
Eating	95
Resting	320
Sitting/reading	380
Sleeping	525
Standing	105
Telephone	95
Typing	125
Washing dishes	140
Writing	95
Personal toilet	215
Calisthenics	292
Basketball	395
TOTAL	**2,882**

Additional Activity in Summer

Cycling to school	493
Tennis	225
TOTAL	**718**

physical exercise on a regular basis would be included here. (Golf once or twice a week does *not* qualify a person to move to a higher category.) The majority of people are in this particular range. If you are not on a regular exercise program place yourself in this category.

4. Add 50 percent for individuals who work steadily as cooks, domestics, and operators of various machines. Also in this group are students doing additional lab or library work at school, provided they stand and walk

at least two hours daily. A housewife who does her housework and has pre-school children to care for is in this group.

5. Add 60 percent for most manual laborers—farmers and roofers—as well as for students who engage regularly in physical education classes or intramural sports activities. Also included are students who dance four or five times a week, provided that these students also walk or stand for two hours a day.

6. Add 70 percent for those who regularly engage in heavy work—construction workers and miners—and students who participate regularly in physical education classes, as well as intramural and interschool sports of a moderate nature (e.g., baseball).

7. Add 80 to 100 percent for those students who play and participate in vigorous intercollegiate or interschool sports, such as football, basketball, wrestling, track, field, or cross-country.

To estimate your calories, simply consider how many pounds you seem to struggle with each year. Is it 5, 10, or 15, or more pounds? Once you have established the number of pounds you gain, you can quickly estimate the number of calories you are out of balance. For every pound you gain yearly, you are out of caloric balance by 10 calories a day. Thus, if you have a 5-pound weight gain over a year's time, you are out of caloric balance by 50 calories a day. A 10-pound annual weight gain means a 100 calories-a-day imbalance.

Simply add this to the figure you received on the caloric outgo. For example, if you find out that you were burning off 2,200 calories a day as you work and play your way through the day and you are struggling with 10 pounds a year, you would be eating about 2,300 calories a day.

Now that you know how many calories you normally consume and how many calories you typically expend, life can be a lot more fun. In this energy conscious age, the horrible task of counting calories can become one of the supreme pleasures in life—you can burn up all of the energy you want to, and it won't cost you a dime. Rather, you'll keep finding more and more energy.

A few examples are in order here. Let's assume that you're out of caloric balance by 100 calories a day. You go through the activity calorie counter (Appendix A) until you come to walking. Select the number of minutes it takes for you at your weight to burn 100 calories worth of activity. For example, if your present weight is 155 pounds, a half-hour stroll at 2½ mph—a nice, leisurely pace, neither very slow nor very fast—will burn off approximately 100 to 125 calories per day and restore your caloric balance.

Of course, you want to lose fat, not just stay as you are. So, select a second activity. The best activities are those that are listed under aerobic exercise. A half-hour of target heart rate exercise usually burns about 300 calories. If you could manage a daily session, you would lose fat at the rate of almost three pounds a month.

You can supplement these activities with some other kinds of activities. Anything that burns extra calories is going to help you lose weight and fat. So the word "activity" as used here refers to anything that lets you move your muscles. It most definitely need not be "exercise" in the traditional sense of the word.

Housework—mopping, scrubbing floors, vacuuming, dusting—is an activity, and a pretty good one for burning off calories, as is lawn work, washing the car, painting the garage, chopping wood, or climbing stairs. However, with the exception of housework, which never ends, as everybody knows only too well, you couldn't very well plan a whole program based only on these other activities. Instead, it's best to regard these occasional muscle-movers as bonus activities. Their real value is supplementary. Do them as often as you can to boost your total weekly calorie expenditure.

In this program, the most rewarding activities are vigorous, and involve the use of the whole body's muscles. Free-form modern dance, cycling, swimming, jogging, running in place, walking, gymnastics, tennis, handball, volleyball, and many other sports are excellent.

Stationary exercises and calisthenics—the kind that have you reaching, bending, stretching, pulling, and kicking—are less valuable because most of them involve the use of smaller muscle groups. However, you can get good results from a routine of several kinds of stationary exercises if you put them together in such a way that the whole body gets a workout.

CHAPTER 14
Strategies for Fat Fighting

It's quite likely that you wouldn't be reading this book if there wasn't an energy crisis within your body's economy. And, as you probably have gathered, the reason for this energy problem is that you've slipped into a lifestyle that uses energy faster than you can supply it. Your body is on the loser's end of a trade deficit—you're importing too much of the wrong kind of energy and exporting too little of the right kind of energy. Your body's energy crisis can only be cured by increasing exports so that you can once again be industrious, productive, and even have a bit of disposable energy so that you can participate in the extras of life that once were beyond your grasp.

You're committed to making that change because you know that, although it's going to require considerable retooling of your behavior, the investment is worth it. The returns are considerable. You know you'll be a winner and end up with enough energy to strip your "rate of inflation."

If you've decided that you want to adopt a more active pattern of living, the best way to guarantee that you in fact do make the necessary changes is to make it official. Announce your intentions to your spouse or other trusted acquaintances. And don't stop there. Take steps toward building an environment for yourself that will encourage you to stick with your fat-fighting, energy-building approach to life.

Fat-Fighting Strategies

Here are some fat-fighting strategies that will make a difference over the
long haul.

Exercise with a Friend, Maybe

We are all social beings, and enjoy doing things together. As you embark on a program of exercise and activity, try to get your best friend to do it with you. When you go it alone, it's easy to skip a day or two. But if your friend is counting on you, it's harder to say no.

Exercising with a friend can be stimulating—for some people. My wife Beth picks up energy by being with people—a real extrovert. Parties, socialization, and interaction are all part of her lifestyle. She gets energy from people and gives it to them as well. So she loves to exercise with people.

I'm different. I like to be alone. I seem to regroup by giving myself some quiet time. With five kids, two dogs, a hectic traveling and writing schedule, plus a fine, fine wife, I need time for Charlie. My run gives me the perfect opportunity. It's quiet time, and the solitude energizes my batteries. That doesn't mean I don't like to be with people—it's just that with my schedule I need less time with people than does Beth.

Exercise at the Same Time Each Day

In addition to being social creatures, we are creatures of habit. Take a look at the things that really count in your daily life. They occur at roughly the same time each day. By choosing a particular time of day to do your exercise, it becomes part of your routine and thus more difficult to forget. It's important to choose a time of day when you are "up." If you are a morning person, try to exercise in the morning. If it takes you quite a while to get started in the morning, do your exercise before supper just after you get home from work. Soon, you will look forward to the time that you have set aside to do your body and mind a great favor.

Pick an Activity You Enjoy

You hate running? Then don't run! You have always enjoyed riding your bike? Then make that your basic activity for losing fat. Too many times we think of exercise as a form of punishment. We rigidly put ourselves through the paces, much like a drill instructor at boot camp. No wonder so many people say, "I just don't like to exercise!" Choosing something you like to do will help you to stick with it longer and see results quicker. Activities you hate become boring. Boring activities produce fatigue or a low level of energy.

Go Long

Surprisingly, the longer you go (to a point!) the more you will enjoy an activity. I've run for 27 years. For 16 years I didn't enjoy it. I ran because I felt it was good for me. Every day it took supreme discipline to go outside and log my miles. Then one day I decided to see if I could go further than my customary three miles. I ran five miles and I enjoyed it. I enjoyed it so much I started running that distance or further every day. Now running is a real lift for me. It takes very little discipline and I look forward to the runs with eager anticipation. The secret as I mentioned before is Long-Slow-Distance.

Dress the Part for Activity

This may seem like an insignificant bit of advice, but you'd be surprised what it does for your mind to go through the procedure of changing into a T-shirt, shorts, sweat pants, or athletic shoes. There's a little bit of fantasy in each of us, and sometimes when I lace up my running shoes, I'm mystically transported to the starting line of the prestigious Boston Marathon as one of the leading contenders for the individual title. I know that sounds far out, but I've found that it works for more runners than just myself. Have your special "outfit" for whatever activity you choose.

Think the Part

Get psyched up! If you go out for a jog or a walk thinking negatively, there's no way you will enjoy it. Picture your heart, lungs, and arteries working together efficiently to provide your body with energy-giving oxygen. Get fired up about the fact that you are part of a unique group of individuals who care enough to do something for their bodies. Take pride in the fact that you are doing rather than sitting.

Do It to Music

If the activity you choose is something that's done indoors, by all means, put a record on the stereo and make sure it is fast. Choose music that you enjoy, but also music that is up in tempo. It's a great motivator. Once, when running late at night in the fieldhouse of a local college, one of the students put a record on the P.A. (public address) system. It was like a tonic. The music came loudly over the speakers and you could feel the beat all through the fieldhouse. I noticed my pace picked up without even thinking about it, and I kept that pace much longer than I normally would.

Add Active People to Your List of Friends

Once you start exercising regularly, you will soon discover that you're not the only one doing it. You'll meet people in the park where you walk, at the health club where you lift weights, or at the gymnasium where you play basketball. As you make acquaintances with these people, you will find that physical activity becomes a common denominator for friendship. You will soon find that you enjoy meeting and being with these people to share advice and encouragement as you pursue the active life.

Avoid Sitting Before and After Supper

Perhaps the most repeated routine in America is this: Set down the lunch box, open the refrigerator, grab a snack, sit down in front of the TV, eat supper, retire to the easy chair in front of the TV, read the paper, watch the news, have another snack, and go to bed. That's a bad habit and one that's conducive to gaining fat. It certainly isn't very energetic. To break that routine, try to stay on your feet before and after supper. Spend the time working on a project around the house or with a hobby. Or spend it with your family. When you watch the news, try doing some light calisthenics or stretching exercises on the floor of the living room as you watch.

Avoid Overdoing It

I had a friend who didn't use his God-given intelligence. One spring he bought fertilizer for his lawn. The directions told him to spread it at a certain rate, which he did. Then he reasoned that going back over his lawn again would give it a double dose and therefore do that much better. So, he went back over his lawn again with the fertilizer. Within a week the grass was brown. It sounds crazy, yet some people do this with exercise. In your effort to return to an energetic life, remember that it takes time. For every year that you have been inactive, you should plan on at least a month to get back into a better physical condition. So if you have been sedentary for ten years, it will take ten months for you to reach a level of fitness with which you can be happy. Take your time and have patience and remember the old adage about Rome not being built in a day.

Look at "Before" Pictures

As you begin to make progress toward a slimmer and more energetic you, get some old photographs out and take a look at what you once looked like. Not only will you have trouble believing that you were ever that fat, you will also resolve to never get that way again. Hence, you will keep up with your program.

Tell People about Your New Way of Life

As you share your success with others, you will strengthen your own resolve in continuing to lead an active life. You may even find that some people look to you for advice. There's nothing better than feeling wanted. You may even become the resident expert on fitness in your neighborhood. There's nothing wrong with that. In fact, it's just one of the many rewards for doing something positive to take care of your body.

Chart Your Progress

If you walk, jog, run, or cycle, use a map to keep track of the distance you've covered. It's kind of fun to be able to tell others that you ran to Hawaii and back. If your activity can't be measured in miles, measure it in minutes. Within a short time, you'll be able to say something like, "I played tennis for 78 days!"

Use Your Legs Rather than a Car

This will not only improve your own energy, it will help to ease the nation's energy crisis. Set a minimum limit. Never use the car for distances less than one mile, two miles, or even three miles.

Obviously, this list is not exhaustive. It primarily emphasizes activity. Supplement it with your own ideas. For example, one friend of mine insists upon eating a filling, well-balanced meal before going grocery shopping. He has discovered that by doing this he is less likely to impulsively pluck packages of scrumptious-looking food off the shelves. Then, back home when his defenses are down and he feels like snacking, nothing is available but nuts, apples, and other nutritious foods.

If you stick with the program, as the weeks go by you'll notice definite progress. If you're like many fat fighters I know, you'll enjoy keeping track of the disappearing pockets of fat. The scales are only one way of doing this. The pinch, jiggle, mirror, and other tests described in Chapter 13 are better techniques. Also, by listening to your body, you will soon "feel" definite improvements after only a few weeks of activity. Your breathing will come easier. Your heart rate may slow down by several beats a minute. Your energy level will reach a new high.

As you achieve these improvements, celebrate. Have a picnic in the park, take the family to the beach, or go skiing with a friend. Enjoy doing something that you've always wanted to do but never found the time for. Even running an extra mile can qualify as a celebration, if you just tell your friends why you're doing it. When they look at you cockeyed and shake their heads and mumble something about how you haven't been acting "normal" lately, just say, "Well, what else am I supposed to do with all this extra energy?"

Realize, however, that there will be no cause for celebration unless you put your strategies for fat fighting into action. To help you get started, you may want to use the three phase plan at the end of this section, which is based on the principles just described.

This three phase plan is designed around choosing two activities that you will enjoy doing on a regular basis. The first activity is to get you back into caloric balance (make calorie output equal income). I call this your caloric balancer. The second activity is to establish a deficit so that weight is actually lost rather than maintained—your fat-burner activity.

A Three Phase Plan for Slimming

No one likes to admit being too fat. We prefer to use words like "pleasantly plump," "a little heavy," or "big boned." The tests at the end of Chapter 13 will help you come up with an honest evaluation of whether or not you are too fat. I suggest that you go through each test and answer every question. If the majority of the tests indicates that you are carrying too much fat, I would suggest that you begin with Phase One. If, however, you are generally pleased with the way you look, but sense the need to drop a few pounds, it might be better for you to begin at Phase Two. Phase Three is for people who already have their weight under control, and want to maintain that level of slim living.

Phase One—The Caloric Balancer Program

Phase One is your introduction to a better-looking body. This program of brisk walking will get your body into shape for the time when you actually engage in target heart rate exercise. Walking is also beneficial to your cardiovascular system. It's mild enough for almost everyone to enjoy. You will not *lose* a great deal of weight in Phase One. Instead, you will quit gaining weight as you burn off those extra calories.

Phase One—Walking Program (6–7 Times per Week)

Steps*	Duration of Exercise (Minutes)
1	15–17
2	18–20
3	21–23
4	24–26
5	27–29
6	30–33
7	34–37
8	38–41
9	42–44
10	45–50

*Spend a minimum of one week at each step in the phase.

Bonus Activities

In addition to your caloric balancer program, Phase One will introduce you to the concept of "building activity into your life." That simply means that you will try to find ways to use your body to do things instead of finding ways to avoid using it. The 10 to 12 extra calories you might use doing things the "hard way" will add up and help you to maintain your weight. Select one of the following suggestions and program it into your life while you are working on Phase One:

1. Don't use the escalator or elevator if there are stairs.
2. Don't drive if you can get there by bicycle or foot.
3. When you drive, park at the far end of the parking lot so that you have to walk a little bit more to get to your destination.

Plan for Slimming—Continued

4. Don't use an electric mixer, blender, or can opener if you can do the job by hand.
5. Don't use a power saw if a hand saw will do the job.
6. Don't use a dryer if you have a clothes line out in the yard, to help you bend and stretch.
7. While you watch television, get up and walk in place or bend and stretch during each commercial and station break.

In addition to selecting one of those activities, try to follow these five suggestions in all that you do:

1. Never lie down when you can sit up.
2. Never sit when you can stand. The caloric difference per hour is 10 calories, which is enough to have a discernable effect over the months.
3. Get into the habit of "pacing"; instead of dropping into a chair to mull over a problem, get up and move around.
4. As a general rule, never sit for more than an hour and a half without standing, stretching, and walking for five minutes or so.
5. Run in place whenever you can, even if it is only for 30 seconds or so. Time spent waiting is a natural for this.

Phase Two—The Fat-Burner Program

This phase combines walking, a target heart rate activity, and bonus activities that will help you to lose fat. The walking will help you to maintain a balance in your caloric output/input. Though you may have already lost some pounds through this activity, the real weight loss will come with your second activity—the fat burner.

You have several options for your target heart rate activity. You can run, swim, cross-country ski, aerobic dance, run in place, jump rope, and of course, continue walking. As you do the fat-burner exercise, you should be pushing your heart rate up to about 70 percent of your maximum heart rate. (See Chapter 9 for more detailed description of your target heart rate.)

Phase Two—Fat-Burner Program (4 Times per Week)

Steps*	Caloric Balance or Walking (Minutes)	Target Heart Rate Activity (Minutes)
1	30	10
2	27	13
3	25	15
4	22	18
5	20	20
6	17	23
7	15	25
8	15	28

*Spend a minimum of two weeks at each step in this phase.

Plan for Slimming—Continued

Bonus Activities

In Phase One you selected one bonus activity to work on while you were going through that phase. For Phase Two, select an additional activity and work on it while you are going through each step of this phase.

Phase Three—The Super Slimming Program

By the time you reach Phase Three, you will be a veteran, one of those exercisers you used to admire. The first step of Phase Three is the minimum goal of most people who are interested in reducing their body fat, because at this step you're getting 30 minutes of target heart rate exercise. This is a very realistic goal that almost anyone can reach. Stick to it and you will not only wipe out your problem, you will find yourself in fine physical condition. You will forget that energy was ever a problem.

At this level the caloric balancer part of your program (walking) can be done at any time. Just make sure you do it. Do it on your way to work, or during your lunch break. The amount of time spent at each step is up to you. You may be satisfied with 30 minutes of heart rate activity four times a week. Your weight loss may be gradual and sustained, and that amount of time may just fit perfectly into your daily schedule. On the other hand, you may want to progress slowly through each step, enjoying continued weight loss and improved fitness. As a rule, spend at least two weeks at each step. Don't be too eager. The important thing is to stick to the program on a regular basis.

Phase Three—Super Slimming Program (4 Times per Week)

Steps*	Caloric Balance or Walking (Minutes)	Target Heart Rate Activity (Minutes)
1	15	30
2	15	33
3	15	35
4	15	38
5	15	40
6	15	43

*Spend a minimum of two weeks at each step in this phase.

Bonus Activities

Go back to the bonus activities listed in Phase One and try to include as many of them as possible in your daily routine. Your goal is to become an active person. That is, a person who finds pleasure in using his/her body to do things. Here's an encouraging thought: When you reach Phase Three of the eating plan and the swimming plan, fatness will no longer be a problem for you.

RELATING TO OTHERS

CHAPTER 15
The High Cost
of Lousy Relationships

Picture this: It's 7:30 A.M. in the townhouse of Jane and John. They have been married for six years and both have attractive careers. John is a bit edgy about a contract he will be working on at the office. Jane is a bit nauseated nothing serious, but she just doesn't feel real great. John had gotten up a little earlier than usual and made breakfast. Jane didn't feel like eating. John was hurt and said something that upset Jane. Then Jane said something back to John and before long, sharp words were being exchanged. Soon, it was icy quiet. At 7:50 A.M. they kissed, almost on signal, grabbed their attaché cases, got in separate cars, and went to their respective jobs.

Silly, right? Almost like a soap opera. But the story's not over. At the office, John arrives rushed and harried. He closes his door, then begins pacing back and forth. At first, he is angry. Soon, however, his anger turns to worry. Maybe he was a bit harsh, he thinks. He really loves Jane and just can't seem to get to work with this conflict unresolved. When he calls Jane's store he's told she's busy with a client. Now John is suspicious. He thinks Jane is still ignoring him. That makes him worry more. He decides he'd better sort through his mail to get his mind off of his troubles with Jane. He opens a letter and reads it three times before he realizes he isn't reading it at all. He's thinking about Jane.

We could pause here for a commercial and then return, but I think you get the idea. John (and most likely Jane as well) has become almost totally immobilized with worry over what he perceives to be a break in his relationship. If we followed him around the rest of the day we would watch him spin his wheels, expend a lot of energy, and get virtually nothing accomplished. Assuming that he gets things patched up at home later that night, when he reports to work the next day he will face two day's worth of work that probably needed to be finished yesterday. If I know John and Jane, it will only be a few days before they repeat their little argument.

You may think this little scenario I cooked up is a bit out of the ordinary. I wish it was. Unfortunately, it appears that far too many people are engaged in the types of relationships that prevent them from living a dynamic, energetic life. Just look around you. Marriage, often thought of as the ultimate relationship, is at best an "iffy" proposition. Of every 100 couples who marry, 35 of them will divorce. Over half of the remaining couples will experience such turmoil in their marriages that they would like to sever the relationship, but feel too trapped to do so. That means that roughly 30 to 35 percent of all marriages are based on sound, positive relationships.

Though divorce is the most dramatic example of a negative relationship, it isn't the only one. One of the trademarks of the 80s is the decline of the traditional family unit. Relationships between parent and child are suffering. The number of teenage runaways increases each year. The lack of harmony between teachers and students in public high schools is frightening. The hostility among the students themselves is even more frightening. And to describe the relationship between employers and their employees, we must use terms like contract, bargaining, and strikes. People are having a tough time getting along with each other.

As far as I'm concerned, there are two kinds of relationships: those that grow and develop and are alive, and those that are in a constant state of disrepair. Both are directly related to your energy level. The dynamic, positive relationship with another human being is just the ticket for an energetic life. It can be a source of inspiration and motivation. Even the most demanding days can be made more tolerable when you know you have support from someone who cares about you.

On the other hand, negative relationships produce a sense of turmoil that merely adds to the problems that you already have. When all of your energy is spent trying to shore up the breaks in a crumbling relationship, you have little energy left over to function as a normal member of society. Somehow, the bounce leaves your step, fatigue sets in earlier, and the inability to get things done becomes a real problem. You become immobilized. That is, because of your shaky relationship, your resolve to accomplish something has become weakened. That weakening may range from mild hesitancy or indecision to almost total inaction. Either way, you are not functioning at an optimum energy level.

This does not necessarily mean that you don't have any energy. Indeed, when you are forced to cope with a negative relationship, you often have a great deal of energy. If you will recall Dr. Hans Selye's explanation for how we handle stress, you will remember that during the alarm and resistance stage, tremendous amounts of adrenalin and other hormones are secreted, peaking our energy supply to optimum levels. That is why, after an argument with another person, you are really hyped up. Your heart beats faster. Your blood pressure rises. You're really charged up. At the time, energy does not seem to be a problem.

What *is* a problem is where all that energy is being directed. Instead of being used to produce satisfying results, that surge of energy is being thrown into the fray. You're pacing, worrying, arguing, fuming, mulling, and sulking. When you finally get around to things that really matter, you're yawning. You've used up all that energy in the fight so that now you don't feel like typing up that report or playing catch with your kids.

Dr. James Lynch of the University of Maryland Medical School has stated that loneliness (even among the married), a lack of sound relationships, and high social mobility can cause a person to be hostile, angry, and frustrated, a deadly group of attitudes that are definitely not energy producing. That is why I call these types of relationships counterproductive. They produce just what you wish they wouldn't produce. Instead of harmony, support, acceptance, love, and satisfaction, counterproductive relationships produce worry, anxiety, stress, dissatisfaction, and turmoil. Furthermore, they take up so much of your time and energy that there is little of either left to devote to your job, hobbies, and other interests.

Unfortunately, things just don't stop with those feelings and reactions. And that's why interpersonal relationships are such an important area in discussing energy. As humans, we often allow one reaction to foster another one. Physiologists and psychologists like to describe such patterns as syndromes. In this case, feelings of worry and stress created by counterproductive relationships lead us on the search for a quick fix. The executive who is unable to function at the office because of problems at home often turns to alcohol and/or tobacco to calm him down. He reasons it would be better to pour himself a drink to escape the immediate upheaval. Of course, the quick fix only masks the real reason for being upset, and puts off the eventual confrontation. It does not solve the problem.

One reason counterproductive relationships exist is because they are usually founded on improper motives. A genuine, positive relationship is a feeling of emotional bonding with another person in a positive way. It's a connection in which your heart and mind unite with that of another human being in such a way that both feel a sense of gratification. Although emotion is an important element, it is the communication—the sharing of those emotions—that nurtures and develops a relationship. A positive relationship involves both giving and sharing, with the other person's feelings in mind. If you would observe some of the relationships around you (or perhaps evaluate some of your own), you will find that there is often an imbalance between the giving and sharing. For some reason, the relationship is based more on circumstances, obligations, the need for approval, or personal gain. Whatever the cause, these relationships produce negative feelings and become counterproductive. Let's look at each of these more carefully.

Relationships Based on Circumstances

Stop and think of all the people you come in contact with throughout each week. In many cases, you develop relationships with those people. You may ride to work in a car pool. Your desk may be situated close to another employee in your office. You may rub shoulders with neighbors, salesmen, and repairmen. While these occasional contacts may not develop into full-fledged relationships, they often present situations that create stress and negative feelings.

For example, I have an associate who rides to work in a pool with four other people. The other day he said to me, "Charlie, I'm about to go back to driving my own car to work, even though it will cost more." When I asked why, he told me about one of the riders that was beginning to get on his nerves. "All he ever does is complain. Nothing suits him. The rest of us spend the entire trip either trying to buoy his spirits or sympathizing with him. By the time I get to work I feel like I've already put in a few hours. I have lost a good bit of my energy."

It makes sense that other people can rob you of or give you energy. In his fine book, *The Art of Human Relationships,* psychologist Henry Clay Lingren notes that "whatever we are or what we have become . . . is influenced to the greatest extent by the thoughts, beliefs, and actions of people among whom we spend our lives." If a friend or an acquaintance is depressed, there is a tendency for you to pick up these feelings. Why you pick up each other's behavior is unclear. It probably has to do with the style of the behavior or attitude; whether the other person's behavior conjures up previous experiences. I asked my associate whether his car pool friend reminded him of anyone he knew or whether he made him recall any previous experience. He said he didn't think so. But a few days later he said, "You know, I watched this person all week. His manner reminds me of a teacher I had in second grade. She was negative, punitive, and unrelenting. To keep from going to her class I pretended to be sick. I was very upset as a youngster. Depressed, I guess, but I didn't know it, or care, at the time."

There is little that you can do about these types of relationships. You can't entirely avoid them. After all, you are a social animal. One of the responsibilities of living in a civilized society is having to relate to other people. Many times, that means striking up conversations or engaging in activities with people who rub you the wrong way. Since we normally like to avoid conflict, we often develop a grin-and-bear-it attitude. That is, even though we may be seething about having to relate to a particular individual inside, we act as if we enjoy his or her company.

Such playacting can seriously affect your energy level by creating stress. And the peculiar thing about this kind of stress is that it's often hard to pinpoint. You may really love your job, but find that one of the people you work with is very difficult to get along with. When you experience nervousness and anxiety in the morning as you get ready for work, you may mistakenly attribute it to your job, even though the problem may be that co-worker. The negative relationship has produced feelings that trigger the stress response and eventually, your job gets the blame for it.

These types of negative relationships cause people to lose control over their own immediate environment. We do all sorts of silly things to avoid having to deal with the relationship. I've known people who will wait until their neighbor goes indoors before they go outside to work in the garden simply because they don't want to have to struggle with a shaky relationship. Others decline invitations to entertainment because they are afraid "you-know-who" will also attend. Still others react by going overboard. They become back-slapping, apparently carefree sociables who go out of their way to display their affection toward the very people they wish to avoid, having learned such behavior prevents any real relationship from developing.

Whatever the reaction, it is not one that most people find satisfactory, and it creates a feeling of impotence. Instead of enjoying positive relationships with people of like mind and interests, the person trapped in a number of "circumstantial relationships" expends a lot of energy trying to avoid contact with others.

Relationships Based on Personal Gain

One of the curses of modern corporate society is called the "social ladder." No one likes to be called a "social climber" but the fact is that a great many attractive societal rewards are dealt on the basis of who your friends are. The young executive may not necessarily enjoy the company of his immediate superior, but he knows that if he wants to go anywhere in the company, he had better accept his social invitations, and better yet if he can garner an invitation from his superior's boss. Relationships on this level become vicious to the extent that they are used as weapons in a great upward-mobility war. In his book, *Executive Stress*, Harry Levinson notes the quickening pace at which young executives move up through the ranks of a company. He suggests there are more young people advancing more quickly to the top in shorter periods of time. One of the great causes of stress, says Levinson, is how the young exec "negotiates the social shoals." In his or her quest to achieve success, old friends are left behind and new ones are picked up that may enhance his/her rise in the company.

Relationships based on personal gain often have strings attached that can be a source of stress. The executive who forms relationships to enhance his career soon finds that he has little control over his social life. When the appropriate "friend" beckons, he must jump into action, often leaving behind favored activities and behaviors. Naturally, it is difficult to maintain such a relationship without a degree of resentment and bitterness. Since such relationships are crucial to success, they create a feeling of helplessness that can flavor his entire outlook on life. Inevitably, the relationship produces such negative feelings that he becomes disillusioned, frustrated, and ineffective. All his energy is wrapped up in masking negative feelings while trying to use the relationship for personal gain.

In discussing this type of relationship, you may think I'm being too hard on executives. While executives may be most prone to this type of counterproductive relationship, they are not alone. At one time or another, practically everyone has been involved in a relationship of which the only purpose was personal gain. Students fresh out of college looking for jobs are told to make friends with the right kind of people. Politicians, seeking broad support from the electorate, make it their business to befriend virtually anyone with enough power to influence voters. Special-interest groups pay skilled lobbyists to mix and mingle with legislators. This is not to say all relationships developed in these areas are based on selfish reasons. Yet it is a simple fact that carefully selected friends can be used for personal gain. When the majority of your friends are merely pawns, even if used for noble purposes, you have put yourself into a stressful situation in which much of your energy is spent trying to keep those relationships afloat.

This isn't a problem reserved just for the big-league world of business, careers, or politics. It happens every day in good neighborhoods like yours and mine. The prevailing question in establishing relationships seems to be "What's in it for me?" The Joneses are more concerned about inviting the "right people" over, rather than people in whom they might truly be interested. Consequently, little value is obtained from such relationships. Instead of honest sharing and caring on a mutual basis, a great deal of energy is spent in posturing and posing to present a proper image. As far as I'm concerned, that's a lousy way to try and get along with people. It also explains the petty jealousies and needless backbiting that often accompanies these counterproductive relationships.

Relationships Based on Obligations

These relationships are closely related to relationships based on personal gain. In both cases, the relationship is artificial. Instead of a desire to communicate and share your thoughts, emotions, and beliefs with another human being, this type of relationship is formed because you feel you *have* to relate. Many times such relationships exist between in-laws: "Honey, why don't you take Dad to a ball game tonight?" Or sometimes you might feel obliged to form relationships because you belong to a service or fraternal organization: "Hey Harold, all the Guppies are expecting you to attend the next smoker!"

If the relationship based on personal gain causes anxiety and stress, relationships based on obligations can become even more immobilizing. That's because this type of relationship seems desperately inescapable. When you were making friends for some type of gain, you may have felt somewhat in control. At least you felt you would be rewarded with a promotion or some form of advancement. When your relationships are dictated to you by obligations, you feel like there's no way out.

Often, these types of relationships begin with a genuine need and desire for positive interaction and friendship. You may have joined a bowling team, neighborhood study group, bridge club, or service organization. The people you developed relationships with in these situations may be wonderful, caring people. Yet you soon discovered that your "free" time was being governed by the group's demands. Hence, every time you left the house to join them in an activity, you felt resentment and frustration. What should be a positive experience becomes depressingly negative. Instead of relaxation and recreation, it produces anxiety and stress. Such feelings, in turn, can create fatigue, depression, indecision, even immobilization.

Relationships Based on the Need for Approval

This is the one that often strikes the closest to home. Who doesn't want to win the approval of others? Very few people actually delight in being rejected. The rest of us will do practically anything for a good old pat on the back. Regardless of the size of your ego, you like to have it stroked now and then. In terms of counterproductive relationships, the problem comes when friendships are built on the need to be approved or accepted. When winning approval becomes the basis for developing a relationship, you become extremely vulnerable to the whim and fancy of everyone around you.

More serious than succumbing to the desires of others is the fact that such relationships are almost totally self-defeating. The beliefs, attitudes, hopes, and aspirations of everyone else become more important than your own. Soon you find yourself saying things you really don't mean just to avoid being disliked. Whenever someone disagrees with you, you become upset and depressed. Rather than carry on an intelligent conversation, you constantly shift your views and alter your position so that others won't disapprove. Eventually, you sacrifice your own self-concept and become totally dominated by others.

Unfortunately, many marriages struggle along with both parties caring more about seeking approval from each other rather than allowing each person to maintain a unique and independent identity. Wives feel guilty when their meals don't elicit raves from their husbands. Husbands become upset when wives don't show an interest in a recent success at the office, or vice versa. Success is judged according to what the other party thinks of you. The relationship becomes a tragi-comic round of one-upmanship that has husband and wife doing all sorts of crazy things to win the approval of each other, and then experiencing guilt, worry, and anger when they think that they have failed.

This is the case with Joe and Alice. Joe always felt that his wife deserved someone who could provide her with a higher standard of living than he could afford. So he works two jobs and even moonlights on Saturdays and Sundays to try and earn enough money to give her the lifestyle he always thought she wanted. Alice, in the meantime, felt bad because she never finished college. She felt inferior to Joe and noticed that he seemed most happy with people who had gone to college. So she enrolled as a part time student at a community college and is struggling toward a degree.

Interestingly, Joe and Alice seldom see each other. As each strives to please the other, they are drifting farther and farther apart. It really won't surprise me to hear of an impending divorce, yet the sad part of this is that they genuinely love each other. What they need most is a relationship—some time to sit down and talk to each other. Then, they would find out that a lavish lifestyle won't make Alice happy and a college degree won't make Joe happy.

The effects of this type of relationship on your energy are quite clear. When all of your energy is directed to winning approval from others, you have little left over for yourself. Poor Joe puts in 48 to 60 hours each week. He's a hard worker who really pushes himself. Yet whenever he manages to squeeze out a little spare time, he's too tired to do anything. And Alice can't even begin to consider enjoying a night out dancing or relaxing with a good book. She's too busy washing, ironing, taking care of the kids, and going to class. All of this because both have built their relationship on the need for approval from each other.

I know this chapter paints a pretty bleak picture of relationships. Lest you think I'm a pessimist, let me point out that, for many people, developing a relationship with another person is an exciting, invigorating experience. Personally, I have been blessed with many wonderful friends who are a constant source of inspiration and energy. Yet I'm afraid too many people exist who are living defeated lives because of the negative relationships that they have allowed to form. I am convinced they could lead more dynamic, energetic lives if these relationships were altered so that a genuine sense of sharing and an emotional bond existed.

All of us, at one time or another, have experienced some of the relationships described in this chapter. Dealing with them is difficult and often takes great courage. The next chapter will show you how you can transform a negative relationship into a positive one—move from a condition of wasted, misdirected energy to abundant energy. Now that you understand how relationships can be counterproductive, you can begin to nurture and cultivate the types of relationships that allow you *and* your friends to live dynamic lives.

CHAPTER 16
Getting Energy through Giving and Getting Love

In the last chapter, I described ways in which relationships can produce a defeated life of anxiety, worry, frustration, and anger. I suppose one response to the threat of such relationships would be to avoid getting too close to anyone. Instead of risking a counterproductive relationship, you could insulate yourself from others and lead a safe, albeit lonely, life. Leading such a life, according to Dr. James Lynch, cited in the last chapter, causes anger, hostility, and frustration. Indeed, this path seems popular for a great many people. Relationships are kept on a superficial level, with little chance of serious involvement. If you ask me, that's a lousy way to live.

There's hardly anything more stimulating than a lively conversation with a good friend. I'm sure you'll agree if you'll stop and think about it. Remember the last time you got together with a few people that you really liked and respected? You talked way on into the early morning hours, yet never really felt tired. Personally, I find such relationships extremely rewarding. But the relationship must go beyond conversation to be truly rewarding. It must embrace love, not sexual love, but *philos*—the Greek definition of brotherly love—brotherhood.

I'm not alone. Dr. George E. Vaillant, in his book *Adaptation to Life*, illustrates this point. Vaillant is involved in a long-term project that has traced the personal growth and development of 268 American men over the past 40 years. These men were selected in the 1940s because they were supposedly the most promising undergraduates of a leading American university. They have filled out detailed questionnaires about themselves at intervals. Then in 1969 Dr. Vaillant personally reinterviewed 94 of them in depth. His comments on how these men influenced him illustrate a very important point about the way interpersonal relationships can make life energetic.

I soon discovered that whether the men liked me or I liked them had far more to do with their lives than with mine. The men who had always found living easy made me feel warmly toward them, and led me to marvel at both my tact and my skill as an interviewer and at their good fortune to belong to such an enjoyable project. I left the office of one such man feeling ten feet tall; but he had had the same effect on others all of his life. In contrast, men who have spent their lives fearful of other people and had gone unloved in return often made me feel incompetent and clumsy. With them I felt like a heartless investigator, vivisecting them for science. During his interview one such man had confessed that he was afraid of dying and leaving nothing of worth to the world. Afterwards I, too, felt drained and depressed, as if I had done all of the work in the interview while he took much and gave nothing.

In short, a person's capacity and ability to love plays a key role on the impact he or she has on you. People who love, have fun, and care, give you good feelings about yourself and your energy levels.

You already know a great deal about relationships and relating to others because you've been doing it ever since you were born. You have cultivated some relationships, rejected others, enjoyed some, and despised still others. All of your dealings with other human beings constitute relationships, but the question is, how do you make sure you have more positive relationships than negative ones? How can you add energy to your life by developing relationships that are mutually rewarding and meaningful? Like any form of self-directed change, it will take a little work. But I think you'll find that whatever you put into a positive relationship, you will receive double your money back.

The First Step

You'll never get along very well with others until you learn to enjoy your own company. Understanding yourself is essential before you can understand others and effectively relate to them. That may sound quite obvious to you, but it is an element that is missing from most relationships. The success or failure of a relationship depends almost entirely on your ability to love and respect yourself. Too many people use their relationships for everything but self-gratification. The relationships described in the last chapter are examples of this. Relationships became tools. They were used, not enjoyed—endured, not savored. Consequently, they produced feelings and emotions that fostered a paralyzing immobility.

I like the way Wayne Dyer defines self-love. He says it is "the ability and willingness to allow those that you care for to be what they choose for themselves, without any insistence that they satisfy you." That simply means that we shouldn't try to manipulate others when we form relationships. In order to love and accept people in this way, it is necessary that you be secure enough in yourself so that you no longer need others to be like you or need them to satisfy your own preconceptions of how they ought to act. When you reach this point, you will be able to love others and do things for them with no ulterior motives, but simply because you enjoy helping them.

I'll admit, that's hard. Being able to accept yourself—everything about you —is sometimes difficult. What about the physical side of you? Your body: is it too tall, too short, too thin, too hairy? Is your hair too straight, are your teeth too crooked, your hips too flat? Now stop and think for a minute. Who's to say what's too hairy or too flat? Are you going to let fashion magazines dictate your self-concept? If so, things may get a little confusing. In the 1930s, models were flat-chested. In the 1950s, 36D was the "in" look. Now, flat chests again seem to be the rage. At any given moment, there is a look that's considered just right. Yet often, you must accept what Nature gave you. You can either fret and worry about it, or you can accept yourself and do the best with what you have. Once you can face yourself in a mirror and say, "It may not be perfect, but it's all I've got," you can begin to like yourself as a unique and wonderful human being. And when you arrive at that level of self-acceptance, you will find that it's easier to accept others. That's where sound, positive relationships begin.

Abraham Lincoln said something once that demonstrates this quality of self-acceptance: ". . . If I were to read, much less to answer all the attacks made on me, this shop might as well be closed for any other business. I do the very best I know how—the very best I can; and I mean to keep doing so until the end. If the end brings me out alright, what is said against me won't amount to anything. If the end brings me out wrong, ten angels swearing I was right would make no difference."

So the first step to establishing positive relationships is to know, understand, and accept yourself. You'll discover that most of the things you want out of life are, in fact, attainable. You'll discover new energy as you pursue those goals simply because you are no longer bound by the paralyzing shackles of fear, self-doubt, and worry. You'll discover life is really fun because you are doing things that *you* want to do, not wasting your time and energy chasing other peoples' expectations. There's another added attraction to directing your own life: those who get the most approval are usually those who never seek it out.

Stand up and Be Noticed

One of the major causes of those negative relationships described in the previous chapter was people who refused to assert themselves. I'm sure there have been many times when you wanted to disagree with someone or wanted to decline a social invitation. But you kept quiet because you didn't want to rock the boat. That type of behavior can lead to complete dominance of yourself by others. Perhaps your lack of energy is really due to the psychological halter that you're wearing, with everyone else leading you around and making your choices for you.

It's one thing to know and accept yourself. It's another thing to stand up for what you believe is right. Yet a healthy relationship is built on open and honest sharing. There's nothing wrong with you if your spouse doesn't agree with an idea you have. It's perfectly okay to tell your friends you'd just as soon not join them for a drink after work. Too many times we give away our freedom because we're more concerned about what others think than what we know is right for us.

I've known a lot of people who wanted to start jogging or walking but kept putting it off. They would tell me, "I feel so foolish, like everyone's staring at me—they'll think I'm crazy." Amazing! Yet think of how many times you wanted to do something you felt was good or right, but other considerations kept you from doing it. You didn't want to be teased or kidded about it. You didn't want others to think that you were trying to be better than them.

Your relationships will become exciting and dynamic when you begin to feel free to assert yourself. People who really count will appreciate you more. Those who are more interested in dominating others will decide that they can no longer use you. That's okay. It may be necessary for some of those negative relationships to drop by the wayside. Chances are that you're wasting a lot of time and energy keeping them afloat. It's far better to have a few good relationships than a lot of lousy ones. Once you experience the freedom of knowing that your friends accept you for who and what you are, you'll never want to engage in another depressing, constricting relationship in which everyone counts but you.

Accepting Differences

Learning to accept and assert yourself will help you to establish relationships that give a tremendous amount of satisfaction. Learning to accept others, even if they hold different beliefs or values, will help even more. You will find that you're not limited to a certain group of people when it comes to choosing friends. Moreover, you will find it easier to relate on an informal basis with the various people that you come in contact with.

There are two possible reactions to individual differences. You can either resist and fear them or accept and use them. By now, you've learned that fear and resistance are low-energy terms. You can't possibly be on top of things if you are gripped with an attitude that restricts you. I've known people who choose friends much like they check out a used car. They're so concerned about the faults that they never really develop a relationship. They're too busy making sure that the other guy fits into their own little value structure to see the potential of a good relationship.

On the other hand, there's a great deal of freedom that comes with letting go of the burdensome belief that everyone else should be just like you. When we give up this unrealistic assumption, we become free to allow others to be who they really are rather than enslave ourselves to the vain hope that they will be like us. When we truly believe it's all right for people to be different, we will stop developing relationships characterized by comparing, judging, disapproving, and manipulating.

Frankly, I find it supremely boring to constantly be around people who think and act just like me. Some of my closest friends are people who don't vote the same way I do, don't worship the same way I do, don't look the same way I look, and don't live the same way I live. Yet our relationships thrive on the insights and information that we can offer each other. I look forward to sharing with them. I am stimulated by our conversations. I am energized by our friendship.

Why people of different persuasions are stimulated and enjoy each other is an interesting phenomenon. After studying human relationships carefully, Eliot Chapple, an anthropologist, has concluded that we all have inherent rhythms in many human actions, including conversation. This means that people may be attracted to one another in conversation not just by the content of their talk but by the conversation rhythms. For example, if you are constantly interrupted by an acquaintance as you are speaking, your innate rhythms are dropped, regardless of how much you agree or disagree. Conversely, if you and a friend share mutual rhythms, the conversation will be stimulating, exciting, and energizing. I am sure, of course, that a conversation is stimulating to you if you find your counterpart to be intellectually exciting. But perhaps the excitement generated may be due to physiological rhythms.

Resolving Conflicts

Sometimes, even in the finest relationships, confrontation and conflict are necessary. In fact, they're essential. When there is a difference that needs to be hammered out, avoiding a confrontation is dishonest and builds a barrier. Eventually, this easy-way-out approach can destroy a relationship. You let the incident, however minor, build up inside of you. It eats away at your feelings, convincing you that there is real animosity between the two of you. Eventually, you let your anger show, words are exchanged, and the relationship can never be the same.

This happens a lot in marriages. People feel that an absence of conflict is an indication of a successful marriage. So they do everything imaginable to avoid conflict. Usually, they lie:

"Honey, is something bothering you?"

"No, of course not!"

When the conflict finally comes, a lot of repressed anger is released and another wedge is driven between them.

When conflicts arise, bring them out in the open and face them head-on. Usually, both parties involved will end up laughing at the insignificance of the whole thing. You'll be able to handle it in a shorter period of time and save yourself all the worry, frustration, and anger of the prolonged smoldering and the eventual explosion.

Another suggestion for dealing with conflicts in your relationships is to avoid getting angry. Anger is a handy tool for getting your own way. In a genuine relationship, you should be concerned less with getting your own way and more with assuring the survival and improvement of the relationship. Remind yourself that anger is a negative emotion, one that will produce undesirable results. As you feel yourself beginning to get angry, slow down. Try to jump out of your body and stand back from a distance to look at yourself. Or focus briefly on something totally unrelated to the conflict. These mental gymnastics help you to achieve a sense of objectivity and to put things back in proper perspective. If you can look out the window and see the sun and remind yourself that tomorrow it will rise again and the grass will still be green and the birds will still sing, you will return to the issue at hand calmer, more relaxed, and less insistent on being right.

The best advice I can give when it comes to resolving conflicts is to listen. Too many times people involved in conflict like to do a lot of talking. When they're not talking, instead of listening they are planning their next verbal barrage. By taking time to genuinely listen to the other person, you are first showing him respect, and second, obtaining some very useful information. Moreover, listening to someone as he shares his side of the conflict can disarm any hostility that creeps in. If you would take the responsibility to be a good listener during your next conflict, you will probably discover that the conflict itself can be a positive experience, enabling your relationship to grow deeper.

When your turn comes to speak, avoid the usual accusatory, attacking statements or rhetorical questions that force the other person to go on the defensive. Any statement that begins with "You" will probably escalate the conflict.

"You never discipline the kids!"

"You always insist on getting your own way!" To avoid this, try a much more honest approach by stating directly how you feel. Share your emotions. Admit your insecurity or anger or whatever it is that is bothering you. Often, the incident is not what's important but the feelings that have resulted from the incident. Only after you repair those feelings can you begin to correct the cause of the conflict.

Handling conflicts positively is a great antidote to stress and anxiety. No doubt, you will continue to have conflicts in your relationships. As you learn to deal with them in a positive manner, those conflicts will take less energy to resolve. You will spend less time in petty bickering and more time enjoying each other's company.

Give It a Chance

Everything I've said about getting energy through giving love must be underscored with an important concept: there is no such thing as a quick fix to human relationships. I'm afraid one reason why so many relationships suffer is that people are too impatient. We are the "Now" Generation. If my friendships get me down, I'll get new friends. If my marriage isn't working, I'll scrap it and start over. If my kids and I don't get along, I'll give up—they'll be gone in a few years anyway.

Earn Your Neighbors' Love

The Bible admonishes us: "Thou shalt love thy neighbor as thyself." Significantly many other diverse religions and philosophies expound the same recommendation. The golden rule of "Do unto others as you would have them do unto you" is almost universal. Christians, Jews, and Buddhists use it. Zoraster, Confucius, and Lao-Tse incorporated it into their religious philosophies as well. It is a phrase or rule that has done a great deal of good for humankind. But as Dr. Hans Selye has said, "strict adherence to such behavior is incompatible with the laws of biology . . . egotism is an essential feature of all living beings, and, if we are honest with ourselves, we must admit that none of us actually loves all our fellow men as much as ourselves."

Selye is not advocating the rejection of such a wise-old dictum. Instead he is asking that we enlarge on it. "Earn thy neighbors' love" is his wish. Here we use the term "love" as the feeling of friendship, gratitude, compassion, and respect. That is the brotherhood (or sisterhood) of humankind. To achieve this love, the best and simplest guide is to make yourself as useful as possible. By helping people you earn not only your neighbors' love, you also earn more neighbors. Selye wraps up this concept with a story told by a Nobel Prize Laureate.

> On a train over the Andes, between Mendoza and Santiago, I sat talking to a Bolivian farmer, and asked him whether he utilized modern fertilizers to increase his harvests. "Oh, no," he said, "that would only create dissatisfaction in my neighbors. I prefer a modest harvest to be on good terms with them." You may say he earned the love of his neighbors by not trying to be too efficient.

Building relationships that are dynamic and alive takes time. And work. If you're really concerned about developing those relationships, you may need to reevaluate your priorities and restructure your daily schedule. Some suggestions follow that you can use to help you give love in those relationships that are a constant source of energy.

Spend Time Regularly with the Ones You Love

This sounds almost too simple to include, and that's the problem. We all know it's essential, but we still let things and people we don't really care about dominate our time. One thing that might help is to think quality rather than quantity. Many people avoid spending time with their loved ones because they think they have to block out an hour or two from their schedules. A quiet five minutes with your spouse before work can really strengthen a marriage. Sharing a lunch break with a close friend can be better than spending an evening with her and the TV set. Regular sharing and interacting with others is a requisite to dynamic relationships.

Evaluate Your Social Obligations

Take a good look at all the club meetings, cocktail parties, service groups, church functions, and civic committees to which you belong. Are they crowding you out of a relationship with someone you care about? I believe everyone should do his or her fair share when it comes to these types of activities, but I also know it can become a burden. You, your family, and your friends are more important than the club's annual fundraiser. If you feel that your relationships are suffering because you are forced to attend to too many social obligations, gracefully bow out of the less important ones.

Venture Beyond the Casual Courtesies

When was the last time you discussed your views on immortality with your spouse? Does your best friend even know what you think about nuclear energy? Relationships get a chance to grow when they get past comments about the weather, the job, the family, the World Series. In marriage, you need to see each other as real people, not managers of checkbooks, guardians of the kids' health, or earners of an income. In relationships with others, you need to forget about what they do for a living and pay attention to who they are.

Change the Scenery

Isn't it funny how we fall into patterns. You always chat with your spouse over the dinner table. You meet a friend at a bar. You talk with your minister in his office. No wonder relationships lose their fizz. It's amazing what a little change will do. Take your spouse by the hand and walk to a park bench and talk. Invite your friend over for dinner and let the rest of the family meet him. Take your minister to a play, or if he likes sports, to a football game. Find out how human he is. By changing the scenery, you jar yourself into concentrating more on the individual than on playing expected roles.

Have a Purpose in Mind

I'm all for open-ended conversation and nonstructured get-togethers. However, we often get together with others because it's the thing to do. That's not a very good reason to do anything. Your relationships take on new meaning when you have some sort of goal in mind. Instead of just taking your wife out to eat, why not decide to learn a new dance step together at a local night spot.

The next time you invite a couple over, tell them they'll each have to come with a story about something crazy they did in high school. Be adventurous!

Don't Be Afraid to Share Emotions

This is, after all, the foundation upon which a genuine relationship is built. Yet most relationships cover all bases but this one. When your relationship with another person allows you the freedom to uncover those deeper feelings of sorrow, pride, hurt, and fear, you will find that relationship to be a continual source of strength.

Your relationships are, perhaps, your most important possession, so it's important to do everything you can to make them as good as possible. Too many people have turned the whole process of relating to people into a stressful and energy-draining syndrome of ego trips, fear, guilt, worry, and frustration. They are afraid to meet new people and to make new friends. They have become immobilized in that they can't escape the constricting confines of relationships that are counterproductive.

If you're a part of that group, you can begin right now to salvage negative relationships and build new ones. The best place to begin is with yourself. Take a good look at yourself and accept what you see. Take pride in the good things you see and resolve to work on those areas that you feel need improvement. As you begin to do this, it will be easier to accept others for what they are. Finding fault will become a thing of the past. Trying to outdo the other guy or gal will become senseless, since you have nothing to prove. You will become secure in your relationships with others, knowing that their friendships can only add to your life. The peace of mind that accompanies this realization will make your relationships a liberating, exhilarating adventure, and definitely will build energy. Feeling good about yourself and others will fill you with vitality and vigor.

A Three Phase Plan for Relating to Others

Rate how well you get along with the following people. If category does not apply to you, leave it blank.

Assessing Relationships

Husband/wife	5 4 3 2 1 0
Mother/father	5 4 3 2 1 0
Your own children	5 4 3 2 1 0
Your brother/sister	5 4 3 2 1 0
In-laws	5 4 3 2 1 0
Your neighbors	5 4 3 2 1 0
Your immediate supervisor at work	5 4 3 2 1 0
Your coworkers	5 4 3 2 1 0
Those whom you supervise	5 4 3 2 1 0
Your minister/priest/rabbi	5 4 3 2 1 0
Your landlord	5 4 3 2 1 0
Your friends	5 4 3 2 1 0

Rating: 5—Extremely well
4—Quite well
3—Average
2—Not very well
1—Quite poorly
0—Terrible

Scoring: Total the numbers you have circled. Then divide by the number of categories you rated. For example, if you rated only five columns, and the total rating was 15, your score would be 3.

1–2 You probably have too many negative relationships. Enter at Phase One.
3–4 Most of your relationships are at least satisfactory, though they could use some improvement. Enter at Phase Two.
5 You enjoy your relationships and value improving them. Enter at Phase Three.

Phase One

Keep a log of your positive and negative relationships for one week. (Follow the format below.) At the end of each day, read and reflect on the events listed in the log. Do it again at the end of the week.

Plan for Relating to Others—Continued

Example

Monday

Approximate Time	Person(s) Involved	Feelings Produced	Possible Reason
6:45 A.M.	Wife	Anger—some resentment	Tired—nervous about job.
8:15 A.M.	District manager	Anger/frustration	His arrogant attitude.
9:30 A.M.	Secretary	Mild anger	She didn't warn me about the district manager.
11:00 A.M.	Jim	Enjoyment	Had a few drinks together. He listened to my story.

When you look back at your log, try to see how (and if) your feelings are caused by the person involved or some other factor. In the example, you would think the subject would have reason to complain about his relationships with his wife, district manager, and secretary and that his only true friend was Jim. Actually, his wife and secretary had nothing to do with his anger. Both may, in fact, be very supportive. The district manager appears to be the real culprit. And once the meeting is over, he could have a few drinks with a chimpanzee and still feel enjoyment. Jim may not be a friend as much as a sounding board.

Examine your positive and negative relationships to see just what it is that may contribute to them.

Phase Two

Write down the one person with whom you would most like to see an improvement in your relationship.

Example

My husband _____   _____

List three things about that person that you think contribute to your poor relationship.

Never talks with me. _____   _____

Spends too much time away. _____   _____

No longer seems physically attractive. ___   _____

Plan for Relating to Others—Continued

List three things about yourself that you think contribute to the poor relationship.

Put on a lot of weight.
_____ _____
Never really listen to him.
_____ _____
Bitter about staying home all day.
_____ _____

List three things over which neither of you have much control that seem to negatively affect the relationship.

Financial problems.
_____ _____
His job is really demanding.
_____ _____
I got trapped into doing volunteer work
  for my club.
_____ _____

List five things *you* would like to try in an effort to improve the relationship.

Lose some weight.
_____ _____
Take a second honeymoon.
_____ _____
Quit going to club meetings.
_____ _____
Meet him for lunch once a week.
_____ _____
Get out of the house more.
_____ _____

Select what appears to be the easiest option from the previous list of items and make an effort to try it during the next week.

Repeat this process for two other people. Remember, developing positive relationships takes time. Don't rush through this process. You may need to spend a week or two observing your relationships before you can complete the questions.

Note: If any of your relationships seem too difficult to handle yourself, I strongly recommend you consult a professional organization that can offer counseling and advice. Every state has a department of social services with local offices in each county. They may include such services as family counseling, parent training, and various resource people to deal with crises within relationships. Many urban and suburban areas have crisis centers for victims of physical and psychological abuse. Alcoholics Anonymous along with their younger counterpart Al-A-Teen and their family division Al-Anon, is an excellent source if the problem is alcohol related. If you are not sure where to turn for professional help, call your local hospital or check with your religious leader, and ask him to refer you to an agency that might help you with your specific problem. Also, a local community college or university can be an excellent source for assistance.

Plan for Relating to Others—Continued
Phase Three

Daily: Try to speak kindly or offer a word of encouragement to at least one person.

Weekly: Hold a family "pow-wow" where the sole purpose is to keep the lines of communication open between all members. Encourage sharing of feelings as well as petty problems that often arise. Spend some time in physical contact, either holding hands in a circle or embracing each other. End the session by singing or reciting an inspiring verse together. Or pray. Or meditate. Together.

Monthly: Form a small discussion/sharing group. Contact 3 to 5 people with whom you would like to engage in conversation and emotional involvement. During the first few meetings, you may have to initiate conversation by putting thought-provoking questions in a hat and having each member draw one. Forego the usual "party" format of games, drinks, dancing, etc. Use the time to develop strong bonds of genuine friendship.

Yearly: Try to develop and cultivate one new relationship. Look around. Is there a neighbor, coworker, relative, student, etc., that you would really like to know better? In the past, have you felt a little inhibited about initiating a relationship? Reach out and treat yourself to another exciting adventure. Your goal is to allow the relationship to develop beyond the casual stage and into a close bond of friendship.

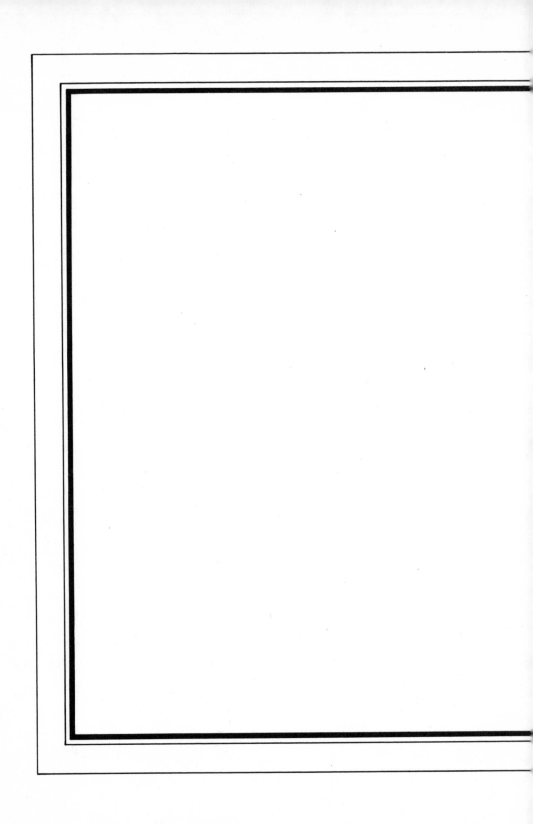

SECTION IV: TAKING CHARGE

CHAPTER 17
Your Life Force

Very few people do everything right. If they eat right, maybe they offset the advantages of proper diet by drinking too much. They might enjoy rewarding and productive relationships but be miserably out of shape. Or maybe they're so skinny they have to run around in the shower to get wet, and yet are unable to enjoy proper rest and relaxation. Certain negative aspects of these people's lifestyle make you suspect that they would suffer from a debilitating lack of energy. But not so. They have hustle and drive, they're getting a lot from life, they are the eternal optimists, and no obstacle is too big for them. They are storehouses of energy.

What do they have going for them? Any number of things are possible, but I suspect that underlying everything is a powerful life force that results in a healthy self-image. These people like themselves. They aren't necessarily conceited; in fact they may be very humble and kindhearted types, but they've accepted themselves. They have arrived at a basic understanding of who they are, and consequently, life isn't particularly threatening.

I know several people like that. Dr. Ellwood Voller, past president of Spring Arbor College, is one. He admits to being 40 pounds overweight and loves to eat scrumptious meals loaded with a lot of things I've told you to avoid. And he is very sedentary. Presidents of colleges find it difficult to escape being sedentary—long staff and board meetings, thousands of miles in cars and airplanes, and plenty of trips on the biscuit circuit. This guy should be perpetually exhausted, right? Well, the law of averages would suggest it, but this gentleman is different. The thing about Ellwood is, he has the enthusiasm, vigor, and energy of a puppy. He laps up love and affection as if it were going out of style. Now, if you're living like that, I'm warning you that the cards are stacked against your having enough energy. But Ellwood is an exception. He's into his 60s and yet he retired a few years ago to manage a gold mine! He is having the time of his life. He seems to gain energy as he grows older. Everyone who meets him wants to know how he became so special.

His strong will to live—his life force—is the reason for both his energy and his successful life. Ellwood told me that if he had his life to live over again he wouldn't change a thing. He's been a teacher, a coach (high school and college), a counselor, a farmer, and an insurance salesman. He has done virtually everything. He still works until 1:00–2:00 A.M., bounds out of bed at 6:00 or 7:00 A.M., and is perpetually on the go, flying all around the country. He likes himself, can offer nothing but praise for his wife, enjoys his children, does everything in his power to spoil the grandchildren, and he loves people. Leave it to Ellwood to notice when a friend or neighbor needs help. He will stop what he is doing, take off his coat, pitch in, and probably work 80 percent of the rest of the crew right under the table. Mental or physical labor —balancing books, writing letters, plowing fields, fixing a combine, raking leaves, or loading boxes are all part of Ellwood's help. No job is too big or small. He has energy galore.

Ellwood hasn't done everything right, yet he has get-up-and-go! Why? He probably is blessed with good genes, energy-wise, and he has done the most important things right. He refuses to believe anything except the best about people and human nature, and he knows he has lived a rewarding and productive life. He has a strong life force. No wonder he has an abundance of energy. If it were possible for humans to reach perfection, Ellwood would be knocking on the door—if only he would eat and exercise properly.

You won't do everything right either. In fact, the chances are good that you, like many Americans, are doing virtually everything wrong. To top it off, you may have a weak ego. You may be convinced that "the force" is not with you. You may feel like a nobody. Disappear, and who would miss you? The political system has become so big that you may have concluded that your vote won't make a difference, your protest won't be heard, your convictions will be trampled. You may have become so much a part of the industrial machine that you've lost your identity. So you try to find yourself and derive your energy from extraneous sources.

Sociologists tell us that this reaction is normal for children. The young child does not clearly distinguish between who he is and what he has. Instead of thinking, "I am," the child says, "I *have* . . . a mother . . . a father . . . a toy truck . . . a doll." He finds his identity in the things that he possesses. For children this is no problem. The question is, have you outgrown this "I have, therefore I am" thinking?

As the child in you matures, you will gain possession of yourself. Your need to possess external objects will be reduced. Having your own crayons will become less important than just being able to color with any old crayons. You won't need a nicer car every year. Getting there will be all that matters, whether by walking, taking the bus, or being in a car pool.

No longer will you be manipulated by those whose only motive is to make a buck. Never again will you let poor relationships drain your energy. Temporary setbacks won't trip you up or turn you loose on binge eating or drinking sprees. Ultimately you will acquire the life force quotient of the Quakers I grew up with in Pennsylvania. One of my favorite jokes, which exemplifies their humor, energy, and zest for life, goes like this: A Quaker was leaning on his fence watching a new neighbor arrive. After the movers had carted in all sorts of fancy appliances, electronic gadgets, furniture, and costly wall hangings, the Quaker called over, "If you find you're lacking anything, let me know and I'll show you how to live without it."

This gentleman knew who he was and felt totally free of the social pressures that plague most of us. He was doing without negative addictions, labor-saving gadgets, and the constant struggle to balance the checkbook. He saw the humor in life situations, and he had no lack of energy. Why? Because of a lifestyle based on a secure sense of identity—a strong life force.

My friend Ellwood is the same way. He is doing more than just coping with life. He has mastered living. Think about it for a minute. You know people like that too. They may not be the "beautiful" people of the world. They may not appear to have much going for them. Not all are that good-looking, their clothing may be slightly outdated, and they may not have particularly amazing talents. Yet they have friends everywhere, always seem to be ahead of the eight ball, and suddenly you realize that even you (who are really quite choosy about who and what you will put up with), really like these individuals yourself and enjoy seeing them. You want the life force they have. You like them because they like themselves.

Fostering a Strong Life Force

In order to acquire the life force they exhibit, begin by liking yourself. Psychologists call this self-love. I touched on this in the last chapter By self-love I do not mean conceit. You do not go around bragging about yourself, drawing attention to your achievements, thumping your chest, or boasting. To do so is conceit. Conceited people, just like those who dislike themselves, evaluate themselves on the basis of how others see them. Self-love, on the other hand, is internal acceptance with no need to convince others of your worth. What others think is of no consequence as far as your opinion of yourself is concerned. Naturally, you care about being accepted, being loved. But not to the point that your every action is carefully orchestrated to present a particular image of yourself for others to evaluate.

Maybe you don't like yourself because of the way you perform, whether it's at work, in bed, on the tennis court, or in the kitchen. If so, stop and think about it for a minute. What does performance have to do with self-worth? Absolutely nothing. Recognize that your self-value does not depend upon achievement. Performance implies that you're comparing yourself to some standard outside of yourself. Are you up to par? Don't worry about it. In the game of self-esteem there is no par. Playing the game as well as you can and having an enjoyable time doing it is the only rule. Don't confuse your own self-esteem with anyone else's approval.

There was a popular song in the 1970s in which a philosophizing participant at a garden party chants, "You can't please everyone so you gotta please yourself." While that may strike you as egotistically selfish, there's a lot more truth in that than many like to admit. The first part of that phrase, in fact, is an unalterable truth that you had better reckon with. Regardless of how hard you try, you can't be all things to all people. Politicians consider it a landslide when they get more than 60 percent of the vote. They don't consider the fact that 40 percent of the voters were against them. They can't. They have to go with their strength—their broad base of support—and let the chips fall where they may. For politicians, the goal seems to be to please the majority. For the rest of us the important thing is to be able to please ourselves by becoming who we were meant to be. Some folks will still approve while others will disapprove, but at least you'll approve, and that's one of the secrets to a powerful life force.

This book is not intended to tell you how to love yourself, build self-esteem, and learn to not only tolerate but actually enjoy your fellow humans. That would be downright presumptuous on my part, particularly since there are already dozens of books on this subject in your local bookstore, if not on your own shelves. But these factors have a powerful influence on your life force. As I have shown, a strong life force can be a major source of energy. I recommend that you consider the following in order to enhance your life force.

Know Yourself

Philosophers have been recommending this for centuries. They spend years evaluating themselves and society to determine the extent of self-knowledge and to point out how much better life would be if only each member of the human race knew himself and what he was about.

Be Honest with Yourself

"Don't kid yourself" is a common phrase in our society. But in spite of the free advice, a lot of us do try to pull the wool over our own eyes as well as over the eyes of others. There is a fear that recognizing who and what we really are would devastate us. Exactly the opposite is true. Getting honest with yourself is basic to achieving your life force potential.

Have a Strong Sense of Self-worth

All of your feelings about yourself are based on this. Until you come around to deciding that you have intrinsic value as a human being, and that regardless of what others think or say, you're okay, you will never be able to reach your full energy potential. This is the essence of a powerful life force— a basic liking for yourself that enables you to make a contribution to the world, your society, and your family.

Be Adaptable to Change

There will always be change. Everything else will change. So obviously, you're going to have to learn to adapt.

Accept Others

There are a lot of strange people in the world. Almost none of them are like you—attractive, brilliant, amiable, clever, and mature. Most of them are stupid, boorish, ugly, childish, or uptight. In addition to that, they might be communists, klansmen, revolutionaries, anti-nuke demonstrators, or snobish intellectuals. They support politicians you abhor, root for athletic teams that you wish to see badly beaten, and even drive Fords in spite of the fact that you are convinced that no vehicle ought to be allowed to exist except for the Chevrolet.

Right. I'm recommending that you accept these individuals and willingly share the planet with them. Look for their admirable traits. Allow that they have a right, just like yourself, to seek fulfillment. When you've come to love and accept yourself, you'll want the same for everyone else, regardless of their race, ideology, national origin, religion, genetic make-up, personality, or anything else.

Think for Yourself

This isn't as easy as it sounds. Everything you know has been taught to you from someone else, whether through your parents, your schooling, your conversations with friends, your personal studies and book reading, or your exposure to the mass media: radio, television, film, newspapers, and magazines. You don't have any intrinsic knowledge. Everything you know has been arrived at as a result of filtering through the many influences on you. So how are you supposed to think for yourself?

Like I said, it isn't easy. But it can be done. The best method is to carefully evaluate the things that you believe or know, determine why you think what you do, and then act. Base your life on the things most important to you. Don't let anyone else tell you what your priorities are. Listen to them, though, because their input could be valuable to your knowledge and beliefs. By being open-minded and thinking clearly you can constantly be building a better base for your own ideas, ultimately to reach a high level of maturity and security, something that you will never achieve by allowing others to run your life, doing your thinking for you.

Seek Higher Human Needs

You probably wouldn't be reading this book if your lower needs (food, clothing, shelter) weren't already met; you'd be out there looking for a means of survival. As it is, you are in a position to meet some of your higher needs such as seeking truth, appreciating beauty, and striving for justice. Not striving for these higher needs is a major cause of inertia for retired folks, housewives, and the wealthy with time and money to burn. They find renewed vigor upon volunteering for work at a local hospital, counselling center, church, or service club.

Develop Your Sense of Humor

The motto I've adopted is, "He who laughs, lasts." Laughter is as likely to increase your energy as any other concoction or formula known to man. It's a great way to relieve tension, cope with stress, and induce relaxation. When something is really funny, people are known to clutch their sides, gasp uncontrollably, and literally wilt to the floor. But a sense of humor entails more than this. It means seeing the long-range comedy in short-range tragedy and recognizing that when you respond to difficult situations in mature ways and with a sense of humor, any upset can ultimately work to your advantage.

Accept Guilt

By this I don't mean adopting an inferiority complex or going around like a whipped puppy all the time. What I mean is, that when you do say something you regret, mistreat someone at home, or make a mistake at work, accept responsibility for your error. Don't blame it on someone or something else. And don't stop there. Accepting responsibility entails doing everything in your power to correct the wrong.

Recognize Your Potential

Why is it that two people coming from identical situations so frequently live in totally opposite ways? One becomes highly successful at whatever he chooses to do; the other wallows in self-pity, never seems able to get ahead, constantly complains about his "fate," and lives all of life in emotional, physical, and spiritual misery. The difference is not in what these two individuals have going for them. Externally, everything is the same. One sees the possibilities in life situations; the other sees only the problems. A cross-country coach I know wears a T-shirt that says it well, "Every hill is an opportunity." I like that. My friend Ellwood Voller refuses to allow the very word "problem" to be part of the English language. "There is no such thing as a problem," he insists, "only challenges and opportunities." The difficulties in life that he has turned into challenges and opportunities would have destroyed problem-oriented individuals, while these same "problems" have made him highly successful. Whether you become a winner or a loser depends on whether you recognize your potential, and deal aggressively and creatively with whatever life dishes out. You can achieve your biggest dreams, or be the "victim of your circumstances." It's entirely up to you.

Develop a Sense of Purpose or Mission

In the decade of the 60s, college students the world over experimented with drugs, Eastern religions, all sorts of voodoo, and even old-fashioned asceticism in an all-out effort to "find themselves." Few experienced success. The reason why, according to some scholars, is that human beings are like onions. The deeper you dig into yourself, the more layers you peel off and the smaller you become. And what do you discover? Another layer. Finally there is nothing left but a bad aftertaste.

To find yourself you must go beyond yourself. Without external goals, commitments, or a genuine mission, you will find no meaning in life, no purpose for living, no identity. You may have noticed throughout this book occasional references to God, a Creator, and other forms of Divinity. Regardless of your personal beliefs or religious preferences, it is my conviction that a powerful source of energy is faith in a higher being. This is the real source of the life force. Joan of Arc probably didn't do everything I have suggested for maximum personal energy, but she sure had what it took to be an overcomer. Her life force was intense dedication to her church and loyalty to the Pope.

Kamikaze pilots willingly gave their lives in honor of their nation, and for their emperor, who they worshiped. Martin Luther King Jr. exhibited limitless energy in his battle for justice, and the reason for his war on the status-quo was rooted in his Christian commitment. Egyptian leader Anwar Sadat and Israeli leader Menachem Begin, though in many ways exact opposites, are both men of faith, though one is Moslem, the other Jewish. You can debate which is right, but you can't question their high motivation—their life force.

The Christian's life force is Jesus Christ. To the Moslem it is Allah. To the Jew it is Jehovah—God. To the existentialist it is a strong ego that gives a sense of purpose in a meaningless world. Whether your life force is exemplified by a strong commitment to yourself, your government, or your God, without a doubt, this is your main source of energy. Your life force is a comprehensive sort of energy that motivates when all else fails.

CHAPTER 18
Getting to Your Goals

By now you realize that you have a great deal of potential energy. The question is, how do you go about getting to your energy goals? When you were a child, no doubt you wished, as I did, upon a star and went to bed at night hoping and dreaming that a fairy would fly through your open window, wave a wand over your head, and make your dreams come true. After all, it worked for Pinocchio. As we grew older, we set aside our childish dreams. Unfortunately, many of us keep on wishing, for our ship to come in, for a new day, for a better lot in life.

Setting Your Goals

To achieve your energy potential, wishing won't do it. You must set goals. When Martin Luther King, Jr., said, "I have a dream," he touched on something that is basic to the nature of all humankind. King took great strides toward fulfilling his goal and never relented, right up to the moment of his tragic death.

You too have a dream. You would like to achieve maximum personal energy. Maybe you refer to it as your "pipe dream," something you never expect to achieve, but something you love to think about anyway. I am going to show you that it is possible for you to make your dream come true. I assure you that this is not another pipe dream. This is no wish upon a star. This is a proven method whereby you can, in a sensible and methodical process, actually fulfill your energy goal.

If you are older than, say, ten years of age, you probably think that your imagination has been destroyed. You no longer believe in Santa Claus or the

254

tooth fairy or even the Easter Bunny. Somehow you have thrown out your own hopes and dreams along with those fantasies. So the first thing you need to do in order to make your energy dream come true is to take a look around in that huge storage tank that is your brain. Find your imagination. You probably left it in the backyard right next to your broken tricycle. Now put that imagination back to work. Let it run wild. Don't be shy. It's the only way to find out those things that you really want. It's the first step toward achieving your energy goals.

Well, what did you discover? Do you want a face fit for the cover of *Mademoiselle?* Or do you want a body that looks like Charles Atlas? Maybe you want to be able to run a marathon, or have the ambition to build your own home, or improve your marriage relationship. It's possible that your most pressing goal right now is to muster the strength to mow the lawn. The point is, we all have a whole range of goals. Some of them are virtually impossible (like building muscles like Charles Atlas), and some of them highly possible. You will achieve them next week, next month, or by next year.

Right now take out a sheet of paper and make a list. Write down every energy goal you can think of. Call it your wish list: for the person to feel like a million bucks. (See Table 19-1.) What do you want? A 24-inch waist? The pep to dance the night away? To be vigorous and vibrant at age 95? My ten-year-old buddy, Phil Lancaster, a cerebral palsy victim, had a goal to walk a half-mile with the aid of his rollator. He trained for a whole summer. It took him an hour and 20 minutes but he did it. Why? He had a goal, a dream. Unsatisfied, his new goal is a mile. His reward—the satisfaction of a job well done and a trip to Disney World.

Put down all of your goals. If your goals are unrealistic because you think you don't have the money, the time, or the smarts (or the energy), don't worry about it. Write them down anyway. Remember, you're planning not for what you are but for what you can become. Put it down even if you don't think you deserve it.

Okay, have you made your list? If you have, you're probably embarrassed. That's okay, you don't need to show it to anyone else. After all, they are your goals, not someone else's. Chances are, they are more realistic goals than you think, because every desire and ambition that you have is probably nothing more than the seed of some undeveloped talent of yours. If you can clearly visualize it and if you genuinely desire to achieve it, then don't suppose that it is not within the realm of possibility. All that you have done so far is to recognize your potential. The only thing that limits your potential is your own self-imposed boundaries; your own doubts. If you dare to use them, you will discover within yourself great creativity, originality, even brilliance. One of the

TABLE 18-1
My Maximum Energy Wish List (Goals)

Emotional Energy

1. _____
2. _____
3. _____

Physical Energy

4. _____
5. _____
6. _____

Nutritional Energy

7. _____
8. _____
9. _____

Relational Energy

10. _____
11. _____
12. _____

Mental Energy

13. _____
14. _____
15. _____

Spiritual Energy

16. _____
17. _____
18. _____

most practical statements ever made is this time-proven affirmation; "Ask and you shall receive, seek and you shall find, knock and it will be opened unto you." But it's up to you to do the asking, the knocking, and the receiving.

Human energy is like money. As you know, you have to spend or invest money to make money. The same is true of burning energy: it's a smart investment. You get back more than you put out. Let's take developing positive relationships, for example. It takes work. Hard work. You have to really try. You may have to go out of your way to do something nice for someone that's close to you. Yet the results are not only emotionally rewarding, they seem to give you a lift that carries you throughout the day. Instead of being immobilized over a negative relationship, you find yourself enthusiastic about your friends. So the first step in achieving your energy goal is to find that last remaining scrap of energy and put it to work.

Warning: It is not likely that you will ever achieve anything worthwhile overnight, whether it be an energy goal or any other type of goal. Everything good takes time. All of life is a growing, changing process. The only thing about life that doesn't change is change itself. I know there are those who say "I can't help the way I am, I was born this way," but I know that isn't true. No one over a day old has stayed the way he was born. We are all constantly changing. Even if you are 40 years old, you are a totally new person than when you were 30, for the simple reason that every one of the billions of cells in your body is replaced every seven years. If you haven't changed, grown, or improved in some way it's only because you don't want to.

Maybe you've heard the old joke about how you were born with two ends, one end for sitting and one for thinking. Your success depends on which end you use—heads you win, tails you lose.

You probably have experienced many successes already even if you don't look at them that way. Don't compare your successes with the successes of others. You are a unique individual. The only comparison that you ever need to make is between what you are now and what you can become. The past is past. Don't let it hold you back. Every day is a chance for a new beginning. Take to heart the overworn but not overpracticed cliché, "Today is the first day of the rest of your life."

The odds are that if you made a very long wish list, then you covered quite a few areas of your life. It might be a good idea to break them down into five or six different lists. What kind of changes can you make in your social life that will improve your energy? Your family life? Is there room for improvement in your religious or spiritual life? What about physically? Is your body in the kind of shape it needs to be in to realize your maximum personal energy?

Maybe you think this energy list idea is an exercise in futility, but it can work. John Goddard made a list of 127 things that he wanted to do in life. He made the list when he was only 15 years old. For him, the list of goals virtually became a blueprint for his life. Some of his goals were rather easily accomplished. For example, he wanted to become an Eagle Scout and he wanted to learn to type 50 words a minute. He also wanted to milk a rattlesnake, read the entire encyclopedia, and execute a parachute jump. While those goals were a little more difficult, he did manage to achieve them. As a matter of fact, by the age of 47 he had accomplished 103 of the items on his list. Some of his goals, such as climbing Mt. Everest, visiting every country in the world, and going to the moon, are nothing short of fantastic, but it won't surprise me when he achieves them.

In my discussion with the very elderly in this country, I have discovered a very interesting fact. Very seldom do they talk about things they regret having done. Usually their discussion centers around a list of "things I wish I had done." There's an extremely valuable lesson here. Project yourself into the future. You are now 100 years old. What is it that you regret not having done that you could have done except for your lack of energy or courage? Whatever it is, make that your energy goal.

Achieving Your Goals

You've got your energy wish list. Now how will you get to your goals? You need to devise a plan of attack. Take out your wish list and look it over. Set a deadline for achieving each goal. If your goal was to mow the lawn, you can achieve that by, say, Saturday morning. If you are 25 percent body fat and want to get down to 15 percent, it will probably take a year or so of proper nutrition and considerable exercise.

For each goal, set a deadline that you think is realistic. Your deadline is the first step toward establishing a plan of attack. (See Table 18-2.)

Next, you need to break down your goal into a series of steps that must be taken in order to achieve it. For example, before you can mow the lawn you may need to put a new spark plug in your mower, clean the old grass from under it, and be sure that all of the rocks have been removed from your front lawn. Next, you need a full tank of gasoline and perhaps one, maybe two, hours of spare time. And there you have it: success.

The steps toward becoming vigorous and vibrant and jovial by the age 95 can be broken down in a similar fashion. How much exercise will you need each day to avoid a heart attack? How much of what sort of food should you eat? What negative addictions will have to be eliminated in favor of new, creative, positive addictions? Then, set up a realistic plan for making these changes over the next 2, 5, or 20 years.

For greater emotional energy, maybe you need to be more reliable and trustworthy at work. Perhaps you need to develop your skills as a responsible decision-maker. Is there room for improvement in the way you treat your fellow employees? If your goal is to go to the moon, check out what it takes to become an astronaut. Maybe you, like H. G. Wells, will even need to dream up your

TABLE 18-2
Wish List Plan of Attack

	Activity (Goals)	Priority	Sample Activity	Sample Priority
Emo-tional Energy			Stretch for stress reduction 20 minutes each evening.	1
Physical Energy			Be physically fit— score good or better on a physical fitness test.	4
			Stop smoking.	7
Nutri-tional Energy			Cut 50% of sugar from diet.	5
Rela-tional Energy			Attend concert, play, or movie with friend once weekly.	3
Mental Energy			Be able to discuss literature, sociology, and philosophy intelligently.	6
Spiri-tual Energy			Become a culturally and spiritually aware Jew.	2

own spaceship. That may sound a bit absurd, but the point is, any energy goal can be broken down into its necessary ingredients for fulfillment. In other words, each major goal is the result of a series of miniature goals. Start a sensible plan of attack on each bite-size goal and become your ideal self, perhaps even sooner than you ever expected.

To guarantee success I recommend that you follow this outline: Take each goal from every category of your life and make a detailed plan for achieving it. What are your daily goals that ultimately will wind up achieving your ultimate goal? What can you do on a weekly basis that will help you get there? Finally, what can you do on a monthly or even yearly basis that will push you toward success? For example, maybe your life goal is to have a greenhouse with plants that are the envy of the entire city. Each day you can water and tend to your plants. On a weekly basis you can do some of the more extensive dirty work such as repotting your plants. Once a month you can buy a new plant and add it to your collection. If you did this, in just four years you would have 48 new varieties of plants. If you're not careful, before you know it you'd have to hire a full-time gardener. But your life's goal could be achieved easily and sensibly.

Break down your energy goal the same way. You might decide that your biggest problem is stress, so you need to start your energy plan by dealing with stress, perhaps through 20 minutes of body scanning each morning and night. This mini-goal can be reached by setting aside the right amount of time each day, and doing your best to insure that you spend this time the way in which you intended. Once each week write down how successful you've been at reducing stress. At the end of each month sit back, read through what you've written, think back over the month, and evaluate your stress level. If this technique isn't working for you, try stretching or something else. The goal is the important thing, not how you achieve it. As time goes on and you experience success in this top priority goal, move onto your next priority. By the year's end you may be doing pretty well on stress, but you're fed up with having to have a cigarette every 20 minutes, so you ditch those in favor of a new hobby —say, playing the bagpipes. (See Tables 18-3 and 18-4.)

At this rate, in five or ten years you would become an outlandish creature, loaded with absurd hobbies, eccentric habits, and an intriguing personality, plus all sorts of energy. But you don't mind what people think, right? Because that's what you wanted to become.

One problem you're going to run into next is deciding which goals you want to achieve first. Maybe you wrote down 20 goals on your wish list. If so, it's not likely you can work on all of them simultaneously. So now's the time to go through that list and rearrange each goal according to priorities. (In determining priorities it will help if you go back and reread Chapter 6.) Maybe you don't really want to quit smoking as badly as you want to reduce your passion food consumption. List as top priority those goals that have the most value to you. Don't throw out those other goals, just put them in the background for now. It's a matter of doing first things first. And it's very likely that you will be able to achieve many goals at the same time. You can take up jogging to gain energy to get through the day, and discover that you've lost 15 pounds in the process. You can even go jogging with a friend and thereby build a

TABLE 18-3
Example of Plan of Attack Breakdown

	Now	Intermediate	Long-Range	Goal
Emotional Energy	Stretch before going to bed.	Compare with last week. More flexible, relaxed?	Compare yourself with a friend who doesn't stretch. See progress?	Stretch for stress reduction and relaxation.
Physical Energy	Walk 15 minutes four evenings a week.	Walk/jog 15 minutes four times weekly.	Jog 15–20 minutes four times a week.	Be physically fit and score good or better on fitness test.
Nutritional Energy	Stop putting sugar on cereal.	Cut pop and cola consumption in half, reduce candy intake. Drink fruit juice instead.	No sugar drinks. All fruit juice. No candy except special occasions. Fresh and frozen food, less canned goods.	Cut 50 percent of sugar from diet.
Relational Energy	Read paper to know what's going on.	Buy tickets, call friends, attend concert or play.	Produce mini-performance in your own living room once a year.	Get "cultured."
Mental Energy	Keep alert for interesting titles.	Visit library or bookstore, choose book, read 2 books monthly.	Return library books, have party and exhibit your brilliance and wit to friends.	Be able to discuss literature, sociology, and philosophy intelligently.
Spiritual Energy	Read scripture 15 minutes daily. Buy study guide?	Attend synagogue.	Consult Rabbi. Discuss progress.	Become a culturally and spiritually aware Jew.

TABLE 18-4
Plan of Attack Breakdown

	Now	Intermediate	Long-Range	Goal and Date to Achieve It
Emo-tional Energy				
Physical Energy				
Nutri-tional Energy				
Rela-tional Energy				
Mental Energy				
Spiri-tual Energy				

relationship as well as improve your physical energy. In short, knowing your goals and setting up a plan of attack is almost as good as being able to jump on your horse and take off in all directions at once. By establishing priorities you identify the goals that are most important to you and come a long way toward achieving them. It also saves you a lot of trouble, particularly if you are one of those people who has trouble making decisions. Now you can just ask yourself, "Which option will get me closer to my goal?" By lining up your goals in front of you and recognizing what values are most important, you can eliminate a great deal of the difficulty in decision-making. You can wipe out some of the stress of life. Perhaps more important, you'll recognize progress when it happens. True, if you don't know where you are going you will be sure to get there. But that's not exactly what I call success.

Getting where you want to go requires more than goals. It requires planning. It requires confidence in yourself. You need to know that your goals are both worthy and attainable. It requires establishing daily habits that push you toward your goals. It demands that you shake off that old "I can't do it" attitude. I believe attitudes are based on behavior. Change what you do, and improved attitudes will result. Instead of leaving it up to someone else, you will start thinking in terms of "leave it to me." The energy buck stops with you.

When a Goal Is Achieved

Even if you have always thought of yourself as a failure, by following the outline I have suggested above you are going to begin immediately to enjoy success. You did relax by stretching for 20 minutes last night just as you planned. You have been losing a pound a week for the last two months by burning the extra calories in aerobic activity. That makes you almost 10 pounds lighter. Things are going better in your marriage because you've started treating your spouse the way you wish he or she treated you. Your goals, no matter how small, are being achieved. Your dreams are coming true. You are a success. Now, how are you going to cope with the new you? How do you deal with this new confidence and self-assurance that you've been feeling lately?

The first thing you could do is take the time to enjoy yourself and your achievements. Celebrate. Tell your friends how much you are enjoying your newfound energy as well as the new pattern of living you've adopted. Rejoice in the fact that you are growing and developing into the person that you want to become.

The novelist John Steinbeck said, "It is the nature of man to rise to greatness if greatness is expected of him." When you set out to achieve your goals you are expecting something of yourself. It's almost like a self-fulfilling prophecy. Have you ever noticed how children tend to behave pretty much the way you expect them to? You are the same way. Now that you are expecting an energetic life for yourself, you are accomplishing it, and you are also enjoying life more.

There is the danger that, as you become more and more goal-oriented, rather than enjoying success once you have achieved your goal, you might tend to become like a Buddist friend of mine who works for a nationally known engineering firm. For the last 2½ years he has been working extremely hard for a promotion. The hoped-for promotion came last month. Is he enjoying it? Evidently not. When I talked to him a short while ago it was almost as though he had forgotten that his current job had ever been a goal. He did not appear to be enjoying it at all. Rather, he already had his eye on a further goal which will take at least 5 years to achieve. His problem is that he has become excessively goal-oriented to the extent that achieving goals no longer brings satisfaction. Don't get caught in that trap. When you reach an energy goal you have been working toward, make the most of it. Enjoy yourself. By doing so it will become possible for you to not only make great progress but also to enjoy your present circumstances.

Remember the words of H. G. Wells: "Success is to be measured not by wealth, power, or fame, but by the ratio between what a man is and what he might be."

CHAPTER 19
The Go Power
of Positive Addictions

We're almost there. In the first part of this book we talked about the stressful society we live in and why getting energy can be so tough. Then we evaluated all of the energy options, from rest to relationships, from stretching to strategies for fat fighting, from yoga to aerobic exercise. You discovered that your life force can make a huge difference in your energy, and then learned that it is possible to reach your maximum personal energy goals.

The chances are good that you don't agree with everything I said, and maybe you're worried that it will be impossible to put into practice the things you do like about this book. That's the reason for this final chapter, an explanation of how you can make maximum personal energy a part of your everyday life.

I want to convince you beyond the possibility of doubt that maximum personal energy is yours for the taking. The way to get it is through the go power of positive addictions. But I'm getting ahead of myself.

We abuse ourselves and rob ourselves of energy by choice—by excesses in our living. We think we're trapped into a nonenergetic life by our jobs, religion, spouse, culture, habits, everything. But we're not. Our problem is that we are living too far within self-imposed boundaries. We are victims of our own negative addictions.

A negative addiction is anything that takes away your life force—your energy—and gives nothing in return. Negative addictions destroy you in some way, either physically, psychologically, emotionally, spiritually, or any combination of the above. The symptoms of addictions are numerous: fear, anger, worry, aimlessness, chronic complaining, blaming others for unhappiness, obsession 265 with money, tension, constant struggling without getting anywhere, fighting life, denying feelings . . . I could go on, but that would belabor the point and it might depress you greatly. These negative addictions, however, can be dropped, and they can be replaced by positive addictions that lift you up by building you physically, mentally, and spiritually, to maximize your personal energy.

Psychologists present strong arguments in insisting that fulfillment, pleasure, recognition, a sense of personal worth, loving, and being loved by others are not optional ingredients to your energy. They're requirements. When you get addicted to things that improve your life in any of these ways, you become a junkie—a positive addiction junkie.

Positive addictions provide their "users" with added strength, more confidence, more creativity, better health, more happiness, direction, a sense of well being; in short, everything you need for energy. Such activities include swimming, yoga, cycling, meditation, prayer, stretching, relaxation response activities, knitting, crocheting, needlepoint, tatting, gardening, writing a personal journal, playing a musical instrument, hiking, weight lifting, swimming, bicycling, birdwatching. One man I know spends an hour every day mulling over a chess set. Unless you're a chess expert he can clean your clock. But he doesn't spend an hour a day staring at the squares and moving the pieces to beat or destroy you. He does it because it calms his nerves. It makes the rest of life easier to master.

To explain why I believe positive addictions are possible, I need to come in by the back door. That is, I need to talk about cause and effect. Take negative addictions for example. A major cause of negative addiction is not merely that people are looking for the pleasurable experience of getting high, or drunk, or just getting through the day. They are driven to it by a fear of failure or rejection, a lack of love and acceptance, as a result of peer pressure—any number of reasons. The negative addiction is the means of adapting to their environment, getting along with their acquaintances, as an escape from the pain of poor relationships or a lousy self-image, or handling change. Although the relief is temporary at best, it is something. That is the main motivation; a brief escape and a relief from the pain. The rush of pleasure that often accompanies the negative addiction fix is an extra plus, or is considered so by the user. Drugs such as morphine can even relieve overwhelming psychological pain, even the fear of death.

Pain, misery, and suffering are for the purpose of telling you something is wrong. At one time leprosy was a much dreaded disease, not because it hurt, but because of the loss of feeling. It has been established that the loss and disappearance of the fingers and toes of lepers was often due to their being eaten by rats in the night. The lepers never felt a thing.

You need your feelings. You need pain. Your sensitivity to injury has saved you from irreparable damage more times than you can imagine. So why deal with it with a negative addiction? Why do or take something that saps strength and vitality and gives you nothing in return? Why settle on a life completely devoted to an addiction that will only destroy you and those you love? Why not rather deal with that weakness in your life with the go power of a positive addiction?

Life for a positive addict is something else. He is greedy for life. He welcomes adventure, change, the unknown, the future. He sees injury as an opportunity for growth. He isn't particularly concerned about what others think or say about him. He likes himself and wastes little time concerning himself with what he hasn't got. Rather, he revels in his own uniqueness and relaxes inside of his identity. He has the power to be who he is.

You should recognize that what I have described is an accomplished positive addiction junkie, and you can't become one overnight. But you'll get there. The thing about positive addictions is, once you get hooked, they pull you up. You get high. You not only enjoy your addiction, you also gain mental strength that you then use to help yourself accomplish your goals more successfully: you gain more love, more worth, more pleasure, more meaning, more zest for life, more energy. In time you will find yourself well suited to and comfortable in this energetic life you've latched onto.

How do you get a fix on this positive addiction, this "stuff" of life? Begin by deciding what you'd really like to get hooked on, something you can do for somewhere between a half-hour and an hour a day, without any need to do it longer than that. For instance, meditating; do it all day and it loses its significance. Or running, which is impossible to do all day every day. You would kill yourself.

Dr. William Glasser, the man who coined the phrase "positive addiction," says that a positive addiction can be anything you choose as long as it fulfills these six criteria:

1. Something noncompetitive that you can devote about an hour a day to.
2. Something not requiring a great deal of mental effort.
3. Something you can do alone.
4. You must believe it has some physical, mental, or spiritual value.
5. Something that you will improve at if you stay with it, but without an attempt on your part to measure your improvement.
6. The activity must be something you can do without criticizing yourself.

There are two major categories of positive addiction, the physical, led by active exercisers, and the mental, dominated by meditators and thinkers. Whatever the method, the results are the same: the positively addicted state of mind. This is the "high" that you can expect to get from your addiction. Meditators try to reach this state directly, by purposefully obliterating negative thoughts. Exercisers arrive at it indirectly—realizing that after the first few minutes of activity, they will break through. Most addicts describe this state as extremely pleasurable, relaxing, and feeling very good. It is a state difficult to reach in any way other than through addictive activities. Also, it is something you achieve on your own, not in a group.

Many positive addicts don't even realize their condition. They just know that it feels good, and they don't want to give up their activity. Fortunately, there is no reason to stop. Their positive addiction not only feels good, it also builds strength and enhances life. The mind flows with the body. There is no conflict, no self-critical interference, no competition. You're not trying to prove anything to anyone. You're in your own groove, with no goals, no stopwatch, no careful calculations to measure improvement, just one mind spinning free.

The positive addicts reach this state on a regular basis, at least several times a week. When in the positive addiction state, they experience a rush of pleasure, something they've learned to crave and have come to expect. At the very least, they've acquired a pleasant, relaxing habit.

There are hundreds of potential positive addiction activities, but walking, running, yoga, and meditation are the primary practices in which significant numbers of people report reaching positive addiction. Interestingly, the positive addiction state tends to elude you the more you try directly to achieve it. The most you can do is provide optimal conditions for it to happen. The addiction is passive. It happens completely inside your brain. When the conditions are right, zip, you've got a fix. When you're relaxed, satisfied, and noncritical, it can happen. Accept it, enjoy it, but don't single it out as the only pleasure in life. The key to gaining mental strength through positive addiction is self-acceptance to the point that you are able to leave your brain alone long enough to experience the positive addiction state.

Reaching a positive addiction state takes time, and rarely occurs in less than six months involvement in a given activity. Some people say it took as long as two years for them. Glasser reports that running is the most strenuous but surest way to achieve positive addiction. The results of a questionnaire he had printed in *Runner's World* indicated that, "about 75 percent of the runners who responded and who had been running regularly for a year, at least six days a week for an hour, are addicted. The two questions, 'Do you suffer if you miss a run?' and 'Do you always enjoy your run?' are both answered with an emphatic yes." Some runners can't describe their positive addiction experience at all, "which makes sense," says Glasser, "because when our minds are totally spun out there is no tangible experience to describe."

Glasser believes that running creates the optimal condition for positive addiction. His reason?

> It is our most ancient and still most effective survival mechanism. We are descended from those who ran to stay alive, and this need to run is programmed genetically into our brains. When we have gained the endurance to run long distances easily, then a good run reactivates the ancient neural program. As this occurs we reach a state of mental preparedness that leads to a basic feeling of satisfaction that is less self-critical than any other activity that we can do alone.

Personally, I believe the same can be said about walking. Along with the physical benefits of activities like running and walking, people are discovering that their mental energy is enhanced and their ability to concentrate is heightened when they become positively addicted to a healthy activity.

Activities like walking, swimming, and jogging result in a great release of tension. It's like having your own psychiatrist. It provides a powerful release from depression, anxiety, and other undesirable mental states. It's hard to walk and feel sorry for yourself at the same time. It gives you a sense of well-being. Swimmers who have been swimming for a few months feel a confidence and control over their lives. It is rare to meet a dedicated walker, no matter how busy, who considers quitting. The reason for this? It certainly isn't the quest for good health. There are walkers who regularly put in one to two hours a day, whereas good health can be attained with a mere 20 to 30 minutes of walking a day, three or four times a week. It must be addiction. Runners *need* their run; walkers, their stroll; readers, their book; and gardeners, their hoe. These are good addictions, and there's nothing wrong with them.

The Flow Experience

A researcher by the name of Dr. Mihaly Csikszentmihalyi, an associate professor of Human Development at the University of Chicago, coined the phrase, "flow experience," another term for feeling high. In the flow experience a person becomes totally absorbed in what he's doing. There are no distracting thoughts. A person who plays a very serious game of tennis may be totally absorbed and have total concentration on the project at hand. The rock climber or mountain climber is totally absorbed in the prospect of climbing the mountain and focuses totally on the task at hand. The flow experience is really a proper balance between the skills and the challenge itself. The person is not overwhelmed by the flow experience. Rather, he seems to be in control of it, and as a result immensely enjoys and successfully completes the task at hand.

This happens many times with exercisers. Athletes talk about the juice flowing, or being in the groove. A swimmer might say he or she has glide. They are totally in sync, having perfect rhythm. A neighbor of mine experiences the same thing while working in his garden. After he gets his second wind and gets beyond the physical part of the activity, the hoeing, weeding, and pruning suddenly becomes a totally creative experience in which he's totally immersed.

There are other people who feel they simply become more energetic as they perform their activity. And that's their high. Not the kind of energy which means they can leap buildings in a single bound, but the kind of stamina that makes them feel they could go on forever, that they are invincible, that they could walk all day or swim across the Gulf of Mexico.

The "high" may simply be a satisfaction of a job well done. A close associate of mine tells me that she has never reached this high and that she really doesn't enjoy exercise per se. But she continues to do her exercises because it makes her feel so good afterwards. "I'm satisfied that I have the discipline to work out 30 to 40 minutes and I feel good about myself and my world." Obviously that statement is symptomatic of increased energy. As soon as you start to feel good or have power it's bound to increase your energy levels.

Psychiatrist Thaddeus Kostrubala has gone so far as to suggest the possibility that maybe an hour or so of strenuous exercise wipes out the influence of the left cortex, the logical part of the brain, thus allowing temporary dominance of the right cortex, or the artistic and intuitive part of the brain. Sound far out? It's not, really. Many times we simply need an hour or so of repetitive activity to "wipe out" the day's problems and allow us to really dream.

Persistence as the Key

The key to becoming positively addicted to any activity is to do it persistently. It takes considerable self-discipline. After really getting into a positive addiction exercise such as walking you'll discover that it gets gradually easier and easier. The idea of a morning walk seems less threatening. Actually, you've just gotten in shape. You're better. You'll be so encouraged by the results you may even be tempted to maximize the intensity of your training. Start walking longer distances.

When you reach this point, watch out. You've reached the negative addiction threshold. A word of caution is necessary here. Like any good thing, positive addictions can become negative, if pushed to extreme limits. The hard-core exercise addict who can't live without the daily run, who experiences withdrawal symptoms when not able or allowed to run, or who runs even when the physician has said "no" has taken positive addiction too far. And it happens. More than one addict has shown up at the doctor's office on crutches or in a wheelchair as a result of the crippling effects of excessive running.

Runner's World published an article entitled "Jogging About" in which the author, only half-jokingly, proposed that Congress pass legislation requiring the following warning label be placed on running shoes, shorts, and books: "WARNING: The Psychiatrist General has determined that jogging and running are hazardous to mental health and present a grave risk of contracting contagious quasirandomous wanderitis (QW), or 'jogging about'." The negatively addicted runner ignores pain, may take analgesics before running, and cannot live without the running experience. Job, family, and friends all take a back seat to the all-important run. Crippling injuries are often the result. Clinicians suggest that runners adopt these unconventional priority systems when they run 70 to 100 miles a week. At this point running can become a self-destructive behavior. The key to preventing a negative running addiction is to maintain a perspective that the running program is a means to an end— achievement of positive health, rather than allowing it to become an end in itself. Control the running experience. Don't let it control you. When it begins to dominate your life you know you're getting too much of a good thing. Dr. Kenneth Cooper, M.D., the man who has probably motivated more people to run than anyone else calls for balance. Running is only one aspect of living. You need time for yourself, family, and friends as well.

It is not likely, however, that you will push your positive addiction to that point, particularly if you adopt something other than running for your positive addiction. You may also conclude that the blissful mental thrill or "high" that can come from a positive addiction isn't worth the intense pursuit. Rather, you may be content to take up some relaxing and enjoyable positive addiction to replace a similar negative addiction. For example, if you are in the habit of sitting down in the smoking room after supper and plowing your way through a pack of cigarettes, you may want to acquire a new hobby or skill that requires exercising your lips and diaphragm as well as manipulating the hands. Maybe you could learn glassblowing, or pick up practicing the clarinet, or potting plants and talking to them, or crocheting afghans for your grandchildren or your poodle, or . . . get my drift? Any activity or hobby can become a positive addiction and can replace any of your old negative addictions. Instead of sapping your energy, positive addictions instill in your body and mind a power for mastery of life that you never considered possible.

The company that tells you to "go for it" doesn't have to tell you what "it" is. That's because we all want "it." You want it. I want it. It's great to have a dynamic, energetic, and vital life. But it doesn't come in a can, a box, or a pill. You can't buy it. No one can give it to you. Yet, a vital energetic life is yours for the doing. Yours, if you are willing to take the risk of being positively addicted, changing your life, and making a commitment to reach your maximum personal energy. So do it. Master it. Go for it!

APPENDIX A
The Fat-Loss Calorie Counter

Low Intensity Activities

	Calories Burned Per Hour					
Body Weight in Pounds:	50– 60	61– 71	72– 82	83– 93	94– 104	105– 115
Bartending–slow	70	75	85	90	95	105
Card-playing	50	50	55	60	65	70
Checkout-counter work	70	75	85	90	95	105
Chess	45	50	55	60	65	70
Driving a car						
Standard–heavy traffic	70	75	85	90	95	105
Standard–light traffic	50	55	60	70	75	80
Automatic–heavy traffic	50	55	60	70	75	80
Automatic–light traffic	50	55	60	65	70	75
Driving a truck–regular	75	80	90	95	105	115
Eating	45	50	55	60	65	70
Fishing–boat	70	75	85	90	95	105
Lecturing						
Standing	60	70	75	85	90	95
Sitting	50	55	60	70	75	80
Piano-playing	60	70	75	85	90	95
Resting	40	45	45	50	55	60
Sex						
Foreplay	50	55	60	70	75	80
Submissor	70	75	85	90	95	105
Shining shoes	70	75	85	90	95	105
Sitting						
Quietly	40	45	50	55	55	60
Reading	45	50	55	60	65	70
Hand work–knitting, crocheting, sewing	50	55	60	65	70	75
Sleeping	35	35	40	45	50	50
Standing						
Light activity–washing dishes, etc.	70	75	85	90	95	105
Normally	50	55	60	70	75	80
Studying	45	45	50	55	60	65
Talking on telephone						
Sitting	45	50	55	60	65	70
Standing	55	65	70	75	80	85
TV-watching	40	45	50	55	55	60
Typing						
Electric	55	60	65	70	75	80
Manual	60	65	70	80	85	90
Washing dishes						
By hand	70	75	85	90	95	105
Using dishwasher	55	65	70	75	80	85
Writing	45	50	55	60	65	70

Calories Burned Per Hour								
116–126	127–137	138–148	149–159	160–170	171–181	182–192	193–203	204–214
110	120	125	135	140	150	155	160	160
75	80	85	90	95	100	105	110	110
110	120	125	135	140	150	155	160	160
75	80	85	90	95	100	105	110	110
110	120	125	135	140	150	155	160	160
85	90	95	100	105	110	115	120	120
85	90	95	100	105	110	115	120	120
80	85	90	95	100	105	110	115	115
120	130	135	145	150	160	170	175	175
75	80	85	90	95	100	105	110	110
110	120	125	135	140	150	155	160	160
100	110	115	120	130	135	140	150	150
85	90	95	100	105	110	115	120	120
100	110	115	120	130	135	140	150	150
65	65	70	75	80	85	90	90	90
85	90	95	100	105	110	115	120	120
110	120	125	135	140	150	155	160	160
110	120	125	135	140	150	155	160	160
65	70	75	80	80	85	90	95	95
75	80	85	90	95	100	105	110	110
80	85	90	95	100	105	110	115	115
55	60	60	65	70	75	80	80	80
110	120	125	135	140	150	155	160	160
85	90	95	100	105	110	115	120	120
70	75	80	85	90	90	95	100	100
75	80	85	90	95	100	105	110	110
95	100	105	110	115	125	130	135	135
65	70	75	80	80	85	90	95	95
90	95	100	105	110	115	120	130	130
95	105	110	115	125	130	135	140	140
110	120	125	135	140	150	155	160	160
95	100	105	110	115	125	130	135	135
75	80	85	90	95	100	105	110	110

Mild Intensity Activities

Body Weight in Pounds:	Calories Burned Per Hour					
	50–60	61–71	72–82	83–93	94–104	105–115
Assembly and assembly-line work						
Light/medium machine parts at own pace	115	125	140	150	160	175
Light/medium machine parts at 500 times per day or more	135	150	160	175	190	205
Working on assembly line where parts require lifting at about every 5 minutes, lift is for a few seconds and weighs less than 45 pounds	135	150	160	175	190	205
Working on assembly line where parts require lifting at about every 5 minutes, lift is for a few seconds and weighs more than 45 pounds	150	165	180	200	215	230
Baking–beating cake batter by hand	85	95	105	115	120	130
Bartending–busy	120	130	145	155	170	180
Baseball–other than pitcher or catcher	145	160	175	190	205	220
Bicycling–5½ mph	125	135	150	165	175	190
Bowling						
Continuous	140	150	170	180	195	210
Regular	95	105	115	125	140	150
Bricklaying	105	115	125	140	150	160
Calisthenic program–low	140	155	170	185	200	215
Carpentry work–light	120	130	145	155	170	180
Carrying trays, dishes, etc.–waitress	125	140	150	165	180	190
Chopping wood–using power saw	115	125	140	150	160	175
Crane operation	120	130	145	155	170	180
Cranking up dollies, hitching trailers, operating large levers, jacks, etc.	130	145	160	170	185	200
Dancing						
Aerobic–low	140	155	170	185	200	215
Fox trot	130	145	155	170	185	195

Calories Burned Per Hour								
116–126	127–137	138–148	149–159	160–170	171–181	182–192	193–203	204–214
185	200	210	220	235	245	260	270	270
220	235	245	260	275	290	305	315	315
220	235	245	260	275	290	305	315	315
245	260	280	295	310	325	340	360	360
140	150	155	165	175	185	195	205	205
195	205	220	230	245	255	270	280	280
235	250	265	280	295	310	325	340	340
205	215	230	245	255	270	280	295	285
225	240	255	270	285	300	310	325	325
160	170	180	190	200	210	220	230	230
170	180	195	205	215	225	235	250	250
230	245	260	275	290	305	320	335	335
195	205	220	230	245	255	270	280	280
205	215	230	245	255	270	285	295	295
186	200	210	220	235	245	260	270	270
195	205	220	230	245	255	270	280	280
215	230	240	255	270	285	295	310	310
230	245	260	275	290	305	320	335	335
210	225	240	250	265	280	295	305	305

Mild Intensity Activities—Continued

	Calories Burned Per Hour					
Body Weight in Pounds:	50–60	61–71	72–82	83–93	94–104	105–115
Contemporary (rock)	130	145	155	170	185	195
Waltz	130	145	155	170	185	195
Dinner preparation	70	75	85	90	95	105
Domestic work–cleaning windows, mopping, scrubbing floors (no pause)	130	145	155	170	185	195
Driving a truck–heavy rig, including getting on and off frequently, and some arm work	120	130	145	155	170	180
Electrical work–rewiring home	130	145	155	170	185	195
Farming–using modern equipment	120	130	145	155	170	180
Fishing						
Ice	90	100	110	120	130	140
Standing (little movement)	80	90	95	105	115	120
Surf	90	100	110	120	130	140
Gas station attendant						
Pump gas and wash windows	115	125	140	150	160	175
Mechanic (car)	120	130	145	155	170	180
Wash cars	120	135	145	160	170	185
Golf						
Foursome, 9 holes in 2 hours–carrying clubs	140	150	170	180	195	210
Foursome, 9 holes in 2 hours–pulling clubs	130	145	155	170	185	195
Cart	115	125	140	150	160	175
Driving	130	145	155	170	185	195
Putting	80	90	95	105	115	120
Handtools–light assembly work, radio repair, etc.	75	80	90	95	105	115
Horseback riding–walk	85	95	105	115	120	130
Horseshoes	120	130	145	155	170	180
Housework–general	105	115	125	140	150	160
Isometrics	120	130	145	155	170	180
Lawn mowing						
Power–must push	140	150	170	180	195	210
Power	130	145	155	170	185	195
Sitting	75	80	90	95	105	115
Making beds	105	120	130	140	150	165
Masonry (wall)	105	120	130	140	150	165

Calories Burned Per Hour								
116–126	127–137	138–148	149–159	160–170	171–181	182–192	193–203	204–214
210	225	240	250	265	280	295	305	305
210	225	240	250	265	280	295	305	305
110	120	125	135	140	150	155	160	160
210	225	240	250	265	280	295	305	305
195	205	220	230	245	255	270	280	280
210	225	240	250	265	280	295	305	305
195	205	220	230	245	255	270	280	280
150	160	170	175	185	195	205	215	215
130	140	145	155	165	170	180	190	190
150	160	170	175	185	195	205	215	215
185	200	210	220	235	245	260	270	270
195	205	220	230	245	255	270	280	280
195	210	225	235	250	260	275	285	285
225	240	255	270	285	295	310	325	325
210	225	240	250	265	280	295	305	305
185	200	210	220	235	245	260	270	270
210	225	240	250	265	280	295	305	305
130	140	145	155	165	170	180	190	190
120	130	135	145	150	160	170	175	175
140	150	155	165	175	185	195	205	205
195	205	220	230	245	255	270	280	280
170	180	195	205	215	225	235	250	250
195	205	220	230	245	255	270	280	280
225	240	255	270	285	300	310	325	325
210	225	240	250	265	280	295	305	305
120	130	135	145	150	160	170	175	175
175	185	195	210	220	230	245	255	255
175	185	195	210	220	230	245	255	255

Mild Intensity Activities—Continued

Body Weight in Pounds:	Calories Burned Per Hour					
	50–60	61–71	72–82	83–93	94–104	105–115
Mechanical work–truck/auto repair	120	130	145	155	170	180
Metal work	105	120	130	140	150	165
Motorcycling						
Regular	105	115	125	140	150	160
Trail-riding	120	130	145	155	170	180
Office work–secretarial	75	80	90	95	105	115
Painting a house	105	120	130	140	150	165
Paperhanging	105	120	130	140	150	165
Personal toilet–dressing, washing, showering, shaving	105	115	125	140	150	160
Pool	80	90	95	105	115	120
Raking leaves and dirt	115	125	140	150	160	175
Sailing						
Calm water	80	90	95	105	115	120
Rough water	95	105	115	125	135	145
Sanding floors–using power sander	120	130	145	155	170	180
Sawing–using power saw	120	130	145	155	170	180
Shooting						
Pistol	85	90	100	110	115	125
Rifle	95	105	115	125	135	145
Shopping	85	95	105	115	120	130
Snowmobiling	105	115	125	140	150	160
Snowshoveling–using snowblower	130	145	155	170	185	195
Stacking shelves–packing and unpacking small/medium packages–grocery shelves	120	130	145	155	170	180
Steward/stewardess work (unless sitting)	120	130	145	155	170	180
Waitress work	125	140	150	165	180	190
Walking						
2 mph	95	105	115	125	135	145
2½ mph	130	145	160	175	185	200
Washing and polishing cars	120	130	145	155	170	180
Washing clothes						
Modern methods	85	90	100	110	120	125
Scrub board	120	130	145	155	170	180
Drying clothes–clothes dryer	85	90	100	110	120	125
Drying clothes–hanging clothes on line	125	140	150	165	180	190

Calories Burned Per Hour								
116–126	127–137	138–148	149–159	160–170	171–181	182–192	193–203	204–214
195	205	220	230	245	255	270	280	280
175	185	195	210	220	230	245	255	255
170	180	195	205	215	225	235	250	250
195	205	220	230	245	255	270	280	280
120	130	135	145	150	160	170	175	175
175	185	195	210	220	230	245	255	255
175	185	195	210	220	230	245	255	255
170	180	195	205	215	225	235	250	250
130	140	145	155	165	170	180	190	190
185	200	210	220	235	245	260	270	270
130	140	145	155	165	170	180	190	190
155	165	175	185	195	205	215	225	225
195	205	220	230	245	255	270	280	280
195	205	220	230	245	255	270	280	280
135	145	150	160	170	180	185	195	195
155	165	175	185	195	205	215	225	225
140	150	155	165	175	185	195	205	205
170	180	195	205	215	225	235	250	250
210	225	240	250	265	280	295	305	305
195	205	220	230	245	255	270	280	280
195	205	220	230	245	255	270	280	280
205	215	230	245	255	270	285	295	295
155	165	175	185	195	205	215	225	225
215	230	240	255	270	285	300	310	310
195	205	220	230	245	255	270	280	280
135	145	155	160	170	180	190	195	195
195	205	220	230	245	255	270	280	280
135	145	155	160	170	180	190	195	195
205	215	230	245	255	270	285	295	295

Mild Intensity Activities—Continued

	Calories Burned Per Hour					
Body Weight in Pounds:	50–60	61–71	72–82	83–93	94–104	105–115
Welding–light	85	90	100	110	115	125
Window-cleaning	120	130	145	155	170	180
Yoga	120	130	145	155	170	180

Moderate Intensity Activities

	Calories Burned Per Hour					
Body Weight in Pounds:	50–60	61–71	72–82	83–93	94–104	105–115
Archery	160	180	195	210	230	245
Badminton						
Singles–recreational	180	200	220	235	255	275
Doubles–recreational	155	170	185	205	220	235
Doubles–competitive	235	260	285	310	335	360
Baseball						
Pitcher only	200	220	245	265	285	305
Catcher only	180	195	215	235	255	270
Bicycling–10 mph	215	235	260	280	300	325
Calisthenic program–medium	230	250	275	300	325	350
Calisthenics–general	155	170	185	200	220	235
Canadian XBX–Level 12	155	170	185	205	220	235
Canoeing–2 mph	155	170	185	200	220	235
Carpentry work–heavy	180	190	220	240	260	280
Carrying trays, dishes, etc.–busboy	155	170	185	205	220	235
Chopping wood–by hand	230	255	280	305	330	355
Dancing						
Aerobic–medium	230	250	275	300	325	350
Rumba	155	170	185	205	220	235
Square	215	240	260	285	305	330
Fencing–recreational	155	170	185	205	220	235
Fishing–stream (wading)	155	170	185	205	220	235
Gardening–weeding, hoeing, digging, spading	200	220	240	260	285	305
Gas station attendant–fix flats and wrecker work	180	190	220	240	260	280
Golf						
Twosome, 9 holes in 1½ hours–carrying clubs	195	215	235	255	275	295

			Calories Burned Per Hour					
116–126	127–137	138–148	149–159	160–170	171–181	182–192	193–203	204–214
135	145	150	160	170	180	190	195	195
195	205	220	230	245	255	270	280	280
195	205	220	230	245	255	270	280	280

			Calories Burned Per Hour					
116–126	127–137	138–148	149–159	160–170	171–181	182–192	193–203	204–214
260	280	295	315	330	345	365	380	380
295	310	330	350	370	385	405	425	425
250	270	285	300	315	335	350	365	365
385	410	435	460	485	510	535	560	560
325	350	370	390	410	435	455	475	475
290	310	330	350	365	385	405	420	420
350	370	395	415	440	460	475	505	505
370	395	420	445	470	490	515	540	540
250	270	285	300	315	335	350	365	365
250	270	285	300	315	335	350	365	365
250	270	285	300	315	335	350	365	365
300	315	335	355	375	395	415	430	430
250	270	285	300	315	335	350	365	365
375	400	425	450	475	500	525	550	550
370	395	420	445	470	490	515	540	540
250	270	285	300	315	335	350	365	365
350	375	400	420	445	465	480	510	510
250	270	285	300	315	335	350	365	365
250	270	285	300	315	335	350	365	365
325	345	365	390	410	430	450	470	470
300	315	335	355	375	395	415	430	430
320	340	360	380	400	420	440	460	460

Moderate Intensity Activities—Continued

Body Weight in Pounds:	Calories Burned Per Hour 50–60	61–71	72–82	83–93	94–104	105–115
Twosome, 9 holes in 1½ hours–pulling clubs	170	190	205	225	245	260
Gymnastics–light	155	170	185	205	220	235
Hiking						
20-pound pack, 2 mph	155	170	185	205	220	235
20-pound pack, 3½ mph	195	220	235	255	280	300
20-pound pack, 4 mph	230	255	280	305	330	355
Horseback riding–trot	215	235	260	280	300	325
Hunting (not sitting)	230	255	280	305	330	355
Jackhammer (pneumatic tools)	230	255	280	305	330	355
Lawn mowing–push	235	260	285	310	335	360
Motorcycling–racing	155	170	185	205	220	235
Pick and shovel work–continuous	205	225	250	270	290	315
Rowing–pleasure, 2 mph	155	170	185	205	220	235
Rowing machine–easy	155	170	185	205	220	235
Sawing–by hand	200	220	245	265	285	305
Scuba diving	230	255	280	305	330	355
Sex–intercourse (aggressor)	155	170	185	205	220	235
Skating–leisure						
Ice	180	200	215	235	255	275
Roller	180	200	215	235	255	275
Skin diving	230	255	280	305	330	355
Sledding	220	240	265	290	310	335
Snowshoeing, 2.2 mph	195	215	235	255	280	300
Stacking lumber	195	215	235	255	280	300
Stationary bicycle (resistance sufficient to get pulse rate to 130)–10 mph	215	240	260	285	305	330
Stone masonry	195	215	235	255	280	300
Swimming–crawl						
20 yards per minute	155	170	185	205	220	235
30 yards per minute	215	240	260	285	305	330
Table tennis						
Recreational	155	170	185	205	220	235
Vigorous	230	255	280	305	330	355
Tennis						
Singles–recreational	220	240	265	290	310	335
Doubles–recreational	155	170	185	205	220	235
Doubles–competitive	220	240	265	290	310	335
Treadmill						
3 mph	155	170	185	205	220	235
4 mph	180	195	215	235	255	270

Calories Burned Per Hour								
116–126	127–137	138–148	149–159	160–170	171–181	182–192	193–203	204–214
280	295	315	335	350	370	385	405	405
250	270	285	300	315	335	350	365	365
250	270	285	300	315	335	350	365	365
320	340	360	380	400	420	440	465	465
375	400	425	450	475	500	525	550	550
350	370	395	415	440	460	475	505	505
375	400	425	450	475	500	525	550	550
375	400	425	450	475	500	525	550	550
385	410	435	460	485	510	535	560	560
250	270	285	300	315	335	350	365	365
335	355	380	400	420	445	465	490	490
250	270	285	300	315	335	350	365	365
250	270	285	300	315	335	350	365	365
325	350	370	390	410	435	455	475	475
375	400	425	450	475	500	525	550	550
250	270	285	300	315	335	350	365	365
295	310	330	350	370	385	405	425	425
295	310	330	350	370	385	405	425	425
375	400	425	450	475	500	525	550	550
355	380	405	425	450	470	495	520	520
320	340	360	380	400	420	440	465	465
320	340	360	380	400	420	440	465	465
355	375	400	420	445	465	490	515	515
320	340	360	380	400	420	440	465	465
250	270	285	300	315	335	350	365	365
350	375	400	420	445	465	480	510	510
250	270	285	300	315	335	350	365	365
375	400	425	450	475	500	525	550	550
355	380	405	425	450	470	495	520	520
250	270	285	300	315	335	350	365	365
355	380	405	425	450	470	495	520	520
250	270	285	300	315	335	350	365	365
290	310	330	345	365	385	405	420	420

Moderate Intensity Activities—Continued

Body Weight in Pounds:	Calories Burned Per Hour					
	50–60	61–71	72–82	83–93	94–104	105–115
Volleyball–recreational	180	200	215	235	255	275
Walking						
3 mph	155	170	185	205	220	235
3½ mph	160	180	195	215	230	245
4 mph	180	195	215	235	255	270
4½ mph	230	255	280	305	330	355
Upstairs–normal pace	230	255	280	305	330	355
Downstairs–normal pace	230	255	280	305	330	355
Weeding	155	170	185	205	220	235
Weight training (does not include super sets)	155	170	185	205	220	235

Moderate-High Intensity Activities

Body Weight in Pounds:	Calories Burned Per Hour					
	50–60	61–71	72–82	83–93	94–104	105–115
Badminton–singles, competitive (vigorous)	315	345	380	410	445	480
Basketball						
Nongame, ½ court, etc.	285	315	345	375	405	435
Officiating	285	315	345	375	405	435
Bench stepping–30 steps per minute, 7 inches	315	345	380	415	445	480
Boxing (sparring only)	280	310	340	370	400	430
Calisthenic program–high	285	315	345	375	405	435
Canadian 5BX–Chart 1A	260	290	315	345	375	400
Canadian XBX–Level 24	260	290	315	345	375	400
Canoeing–4 mph	320	355	390	425	450	490
Dancing–polka	275	305	335	365	395	425
Digging	255	285	310	340	365	390
Fencing–competitive (vigorous)	315	345	380	415	445	480
Football						
Playground–touch	310	340	375	405	435	470
Officiating	285	315	345	375	405	435
Gymnastics–medium	260	290	315	345	375	400
Handball						
Cut-throat	310	340	375	405	435	470
4 people	260	290	315	345	375	400

Calories Burned Per Hour								
116–126	127–137	138–148	149–159	160–170	171–181	182–192	193–203	204–214
295	310	330	350	370	385	405	425	425
250	270	285	300	315	335	350	365	365
265	280	300	315	330	350	365	385	385
290	310	330	345	365	385	405	420	420
375	400	425	450	475	500	525	550	550
375	400	425	450	475	500	525	550	550
375	400	425	450	475	500	525	550	550
250	270	285	300	315	335	350	365	365
250	270	285	300	315	335	350	365	365

Calories Burned Per Hour								
116–126	127–137	138–148	149–159	160–170	171–181	182–192	193–203	204–214
510	545	575	610	645	675	710	740	740
465	495	525	555	585	615	645	675	675
465	495	525	555	585	615	645	675	675
510	545	575	610	645	675	710	745	745
460	490	520	550	580	610	640	670	670
465	495	525	555	585	615	645	675	675
430	455	485	510	540	565	595	620	620
430	455	485	510	540	565	595	620	620
525	560	595	625	660	695	730	765	765
455	480	510	540	570	600	630	655	655
420	445	475	500	525	555	580	610	610
510	545	575	610	645	675	710	745	745
500	535	565	600	630	665	695	730	730
465	495	525	555	585	615	645	675	675
430	455	485	510	540	565	595	620	620
500	535	565	600	630	665	695	730	730
430	455	485	510	540	565	595	620	620

Moderate-High Intensity Activities—Continued

Body Weight in Pounds:	Calories Burned Per Hour					
	50–60	61–71	72–82	83–93	94–104	105–115
Hill climbing	310	340	375	405	435	470
Horseback riding–gallop	310	340	375	405	435	470
Mountain climbing	310	340	375	405	435	470
Orienteering	310	340	375	405	435	470
Ropeskipping						
50–60 skips per minute (left foot only)	260	290	315	345	375	400
70–80 skips per minute (left foot only)	285	315	345	375	405	435
Run in place						
50–60 steps per minute (left foot only)	260	290	315	345	375	400
70–80 steps per minute (left foot only)	285	315	345	375	405	435
Skating–vigorous						
Ice	320	355	385	420	455	485
Roller	320	355	385	420	455	485
Skiing–downhill (continuous riding and lifts not included)	305	335	370	400	435	465
Snowshoveling–light	315	345	380	415	445	475
Soccer	310	340	375	405	435	470
Swimming–crawl						
35 yards per minute	275	305	335	365	395	425
40 yards per minute	310	340	375	405	435	470
Tennis–singles, competitive	310	340	375	405	435	470
Volleyball–competitive	310	340	375	405	435	470
Walking–5 mph	285	315	345	375	405	435
Water skiing	245	275	300	325	350	375

High Intensity Activities

Body Weight in Pounds:	Calories Burned Per Hour					
	50–60	61–71	72–82	83–93	94–104	105–115
Basketball–game (full court, continuous)	385	425	465	505	545	585
Bicycling–13 mph	335	370	410	445	480	515
Canadian 5BX–Chart 2A	330	365	400	435	470	505

			Calories Burned Per Hour					
116–126	127–137	138–148	149–159	160–170	171–181	182–192	193–203	204–214
500	535	565	600	630	665	695	730	730
500	535	565	600	630	665	695	730	730
500	535	565	600	630	665	695	730	730
500	535	565	600	630	665	695	730	730
430	455	485	510	540	565	595	620	620
465	495	525	555	585	615	645	675	675
430	455	485	510	540	565	595	620	620
465	495	525	555	585	615	645	675	675
520	555	590	620	655	690	720	755	755
520	555	590	620	655	690	720	755	755
500	530	560	595	625	660	690	720	720
510	545	575	610	645	675	710	745	745
500	535	565	600	630	665	695	730	730
455	480	510	540	570	600	630	655	655
500	535	565	600	630	665	695	730	730
500	535	565	600	630	665	695	730	730
500	535	565	600	630	665	695	730	730
465	495	525	555	585	615	645	675	675
405	430	455	480	505	535	560	585	585

			Calories Burned Per Hour					
116–126	127–137	138–148	149–159	160–170	171–181	182–192	193–203	204–214
630	670	710	750	790	830	870	910	910
550	585	620	655	690	725	760	795	795
540	575	610	645	680	715	750	785	785

High Intensity Activities—Continued

Body Weight in Pounds:	Calories Burned Per Hour					
	50–60	61–71	72–82	83–93	94–104	105–115
Canadian XBX						
Level 36	335	370	410	445	480	515
Level 48	405	450	490	535	575	620
Dancing–aerobic (high)	335	370	405	445	480	515
Gymnastics–hard	365	405	440	480	520	555
Handball–2 people	400	440	485	525	565	610
Jogging–5.5 mph	335	370	405	445	480	515
Judo	405	450	490	535	575	620
Karate	405	450	490	535	575	620
Martial arts	405	450	490	535	575	620
Ropeskipping–90–100 skips per minute (left foot only)	335	370	405	445	480	515
Rowing–vigorous, 4 mph	335	370	405	445	480	515
Rowing machine–vigorous	335	370	405	445	480	515
Run in place–90–100 steps per minute (left foot only)	335	370	405	445	480	515
Running						
5.5 mph	335	370	405	445	480	515
7.2 mph	360	395	435	475	510	550
Skiing–cross-country, 5 mph	360	395	435	475	510	550
Stationary bicycle (resistance sufficient to get pulse rate to 130)–15 mph	335	370	405	445	480	515
Swimming–crawl, 45 yards per minute	355	390	430	465	500	540
Trampolining	405	450	490	535	575	620
Treadmill–5.5 mph	335	370	405	445	480	515
Walking–5.5 mph	335	370	405	445	480	515

Very High Intensity Activities

Body Weight in Pounds:	Calories Burned Per Hour					
	50–60	61–71	72–82	83–93	94–104	105–115
Bench stepping–30 steps per minute						
12 inches	410	455	495	540	585	625
16 inches	570	630	690	750	810	870
18 inches	720	795	870	945	1020	1095

Calories Burned Per Hour								
116–126	127–137	138–148	149–159	160–170	171–181	182–192	193–203	204–214
550	585	620	655	690	725	760	795	795
660	705	750	790	835	875	920	960	960
550	585	620	655	690	725	760	795	795
595	635	670	710	750	785	825	865	865
650	695	735	775	820	860	905	945	945
550	585	620	655	690	725	760	795	795
660	705	750	790	835	875	920	960	960
660	705	750	790	835	875	920	960	960
660	705	750	790	835	875	920	960	960
550	585	620	655	690	725	760	795	795
550	585	620	655	690	725	760	795	795
550	585	620	655	690	725	760	795	795
550	585	620	655	690	725	760	795	795
550	585	620	655	690	725	760	795	795
585	625	660	700	735	775	810	850	850
585	625	660	700	735	775	810	850	850
550	585	620	655	690	725	760	795	795
575	615	650	690	725	765	800	835	835
660	705	750	790	835	875	920	960	960
550	585	620	655	690	725	760	795	795
550	585	620	655	690	725	760	795	795

Calories Burned Per Hour								
116–126	127–137	138–148	149–159	160–170	171–181	182–192	193–203	204–214
670	715	755	800	840	885	930	970	970
930	990	1050	1100	1170	1230	1290	1350	1350
1170	1245	1325	1400	1475	1550	1625	1700	1700

Very High Intensity Activities—Continued

Body Weight in Pounds:	Calories Burned Per Hour					
	50–60	61–71	72–82	83–93	94–104	105–115
Canadian 5BX						
Charts 3A & 4A	495	545	600	650	700	755
Charts 5A & 6A	500	550	600	655	705	760
Football–tackle	430	475	520	565	610	660
Hockey						
Ice	460	510	560	610	655	705
Field	460	510	560	610	655	705
Lacrosse	460	510	560	610	655	705
Ropeskipping						
110–120 skips per minute (left foot only)	460	510	560	610	655	705
130–140 skips per minute (left foot only)	615	680	745	810	875	940
Run in place						
110–120 steps per minute (left foot only)	460	510	560	610	655	705
130–140 steps per minute (left foot only)	615	680	745	810	875	940
Running						
8 mph	410	455	495	540	585	625
8.7 mph	460	510	560	610	655	705
11.4 mph	625	695	760	825	890	955
12.5 mph	800	880	965	1050	1135	1220
Skiing–cross country, 9 mph	515	565	620	675	730	785
Snowshoveling–heavy	540	600	655	710	770	825
Sprinting	1255	1385	1520	1650	1780	1915
Stationary bicycle (resistance sufficient to get pulse rate to 130)–20 mph	455	505	550	600	650	700
Swimming–crawl, 55 yards per minute	430	475	520	565	610	660
Treadmill						
7.2 mph	410	455	495	540	585	625
8 mph	460	510	560	610	655	705
Walking–upstairs, 2 at a time, rapidly	515	565	620	675	730	785

Calories Burned Per Hour								
116–126	127–137	138–148	149–159	160–170	171–181	182–192	193–203	204–214
805	855	910	960	1010	1065	1115	1170	1170
810	865	915	970	1020	1075	1125	1180	1180
705	750	795	835	885	930	975	1020	1020
755	805	850	900	950	1000	1045	1095	1095
755	805	850	900	950	1000	1045	1095	1095
755	805	850	900	950	1000	1045	1095	1095
755	805	850	900	950	1000	1045	1095	1095
1005	1070	1135	1200	1265	1330	1395	1460	1460
755	805	850	900	950	1000	1045	1095	1095
1005	1070	1135	1200	1265	1330	1395	1460	1460
670	715	755	800	845	885	930	975	975
755	805	850	900	950	1000	1045	1095	1095
1025	1090	1155	1220	1285	1355	1420	1485	1485
1300	1385	1470	1555	1640	1720	1805	1890	1890
835	890	945	1000	1055	1105	1160	1215	1215
885	940	995	1055	1110	1170	1225	1280	1280
2045	2180	2310	2440	2575	2705	2840	2970	2970
745	795	840	885	935	985	1030	1080	1080
705	750	795	835	885	930	975	1020	1020
670	715	755	800	845	885	930	975	975
755	805	850	900	950	1000	1045	1095	1095
835	890	945	1000	1055	1105	1160	1215	1215

APPENDIX B
Calorie Content of Food

Food	Amount	Calories
Apple	1 small	100
Apple Cider	¾ cup	75
Apple Pie	Average piece	400
Applesauce, Canned	½ cup	50
Apricots	5 medium	95
Asparagus	12 stalks	25
Avocado	1 small	425
Bacon, Fried	3 strips, crisp	100
Banana	1 medium	100
Barbecued Spareribs	6 average ribs	350
Beans, Baked	1 cup	200
Beans, String	1 cup	25
Beef Bouillon	1 cup	25
Beef, Filet Mignon	Average serving	250
Beef Roast	Average serving	200
Beef, Swiss Steak	1½ ounces	150
Beer	12 ounces	150
Beets	½ cup	35
Biscuit, Buttermilk	2 small or 1 large	110
Blueberries, Fresh	1 cup	100
Blueberry Pie	Average piece	375
Bologna	2 ounces	125
Bourbon	1 shot	100
Brandy	1 shot	75
Bread, Corn	2-inch square	200
Bread, White	1 slice	65
Bread, Whole Wheat	1 slice	65
Broccoli	1 cup	45
Brownies	2-inch square	150
Butter	Average pat	40
Buttermilk	1 cup	85
Cabbage, Green, Boiled	1 cup	40
Cake, Chocolate	Average serving	250
Cake, Sponge	Average piece	125
Cantaloupe	½ medium	50
Carbonated Beverages	1 average	75
Carrots, Raw	1 medium	25
Catsup	1 tablespoon	25
Champagne, Domestic	1 glass	85
Cheese, American	1 slice	100
Cheesecake	Average slice	350
Cheese, Cheddar	1½ ounces	150
Cherry Pie	Average piece	350
Chewing Gum	1 stick	6
Chicken, Barbecued	Average serving	200
Chicken, Fried	Average serving	325

Appendix B—Continued

Food	Amount	Calories
Chicken, Roasted	Average serving	250
Chicken Salad	Average serving	225
Chili Con Carne	½ cup	250
Chocolate Bar	Average	250
Chocolate Chip Cookies	3 small	65
Chocolate Milk	1 cup	225
Chop Suey, Beef	½ cup	275
Cinnamon Toast	1 slice	200
Clam Chowder, New England	Average portion	225
Coffee, Black	1 cup	0
Coffee with Cream	1 tablespoon cream	30
Coffee with Sugar	1 teaspoon sugar	18
Cola	6 ounces	75
Cole Slaw	6 ounces	20
Corn Flakes	1 ounce or 1 cup	100
Corn, Fresh Frozen	1 cup	140
Corn Oil	1 tablespoon	120
Corned Beef Hash	½ cup	150
Cottage Cheese	1 cup	215
Crackers, Saltines	6 2-inch squares	100
Cream Cheese	1 tablespoon	50
Cucumber	1 8-inch	20
Cupcake	1 small	100
Custard	½ cup	125
Daiquiri	1 cocktail	125
Doughnut	Average	150
Dressing, Thousand Island	1 tablespoon	100
Egg	1 average	75
Egg, Fried	1 average	100
English Muffin	1 average	150
Fish, Tuna, Canned in Oil	½ cup	250
Frankfurter	1	125
French Onion Soup with Croutons	1 cup	150
Fruit Cocktail, Canned	Average serving	100
Fruit Jam	1 tablespoon	50
Gin	2 ounces	150
Goulash, Hungarian	Average serving	350
Grapefruit	½ small	50
Haddock, Baked	Average serving	180
Ham, Baked	Average slice	350
Ham, Smoked	Average serving	450
Hamburger, Broiled	2-ounce patty	200
Hamburger, Fried	2-ounce patty	225
Honey	1 tablespoon	65
Hot Fudge Sundae	Average serving	400
Ice Cream, All Flavors	Average scoop	150

Appendix B—Continued

Food	Amount	Calories
Lamb Chop, Broiled	1-inch thick	250
Lamb Roast	Average serving	200
Lemonade	1 cup	100
Lentil Soup	1 cup	300
Liver, Beef	Average serving	150
Lox	2 ounces	200
Macaroni and Cheese	½ cup	225
Malted Milk, with Ice Cream	1	400
Manhattan	1 cocktail	175
Margarine	1 tablespoon	100
Martini	1 cocktail	125
Mayonnaise	1 tablespoon	100
Meat Loaf	Average serving	225
Milk, Whole	¾ cup	125
Muffin, Blueberry	1 average	110
Mushroom Pizza	⅙ 12-inch diameter	200
Mushroom Soup, Creamed	1 cup	200
Nectarine	1 medium	50
Noodle Soup	1 cup	125
Oatmeal, Cooked	½ cup	75
Omelet	2 eggs, 1 teaspoon butter	185
Omelet, Western	Average	325
Orange	1 medium	75
Orange Juice	6 ounces	75
Oyster Stew with Milk	1 cup	200
Oysters, on the Half Shell	6 medium	50
Pancakes, with 2 Teaspoons Butter, 2 Tablespoons Syrup	3 (4-inch diameter)	470
Peach, Fresh	1 medium	50
Peaches, Canned in Syrup	2 halves	125
Peanut Butter	1 tablespoon	100
Peanuts	10	100
Pineapple, Canned	1 slice	75
Pineapple Upside-Down Cake	Average piece	250
Popcorn, Plain	1 cup	50
Pork Chop, Broiled	1 medium	225
Pork Chop, Fried	1 medium	250
Pork Roast	Average serving	200
Potato, Baked	1 medium	125
Potato, Boiled	1 medium	150
Potato Chips	½ cup	100
Potato, French Fried	6 average	100
Potato, Hashed Brown	1 medium	225
Potato, Mashed with 1 Teaspoon Butter and 2 Tablespoons Milk	1 medium	180
Pound Cake	Average slice	125

Appendix B—Continued

Food	Amount	Calories
Pretzels	6 average	100
Pumpkin Pie	Average piece	325
Raisins, Seeded	½ cup	225
Red Wine	1 glass	75
Rice, Boiled, White	¾ cup	100
Roll, Plain	1 small	75
Rum, Bacardi	1½ ounces	100
Salmon, Baked	1 serving	250
Sardines, Canned	4	100
Sausage, Pork	2 3-inch links	150
Scotch	1 shot	100
Sherbet, Fruit-Flavored	Average scoop	100
Shortcake, Strawberry	Average serving	350
Shrimp	10 average	100
Skim Milk	1 cup	85
Soup, Bean	1 cup	225
Soup, Chicken Noodle	1 cup	125
Soup, Mushroom, Creamed	1 cup	200
Soup, Tomato	1 cup	100
Soup, Vegetable	1 cup	100
Spaghetti with Meat Sauce	4 ounces	275
Spinach	½ cup	25
Squash, Winter, Baked, Mashed	8 ounces	100
Stew, Beef	1 cup	250
Strawberries, Fresh	1 cup	50
Stroganoff, Beef	Average serving	350
Sugar, Granulated	1 teaspoon	18
Sweet Potato, Canned	1 cup	235
Sweet Roll	Average	125
Tomato, Fresh	1 medium	25
Tomato Juice	1 cup	50
Turkey	Average serving	175
Veal Cutlet, Broiled	Average serving	125
Vodka	1 ounce	125
Waffle	1	225
White Wine	1 glass	135
Yogurt	1 cup	165

References for
Three Phase Energy Plans

Selected References for Three Phase Plan for Enjoying Life

Phase I

Cannon, W. B. *The Wisdom of the Body.* New York, NY: W. W. Norton and Co., 1932.

Friedman, M., and Rosenman, R. *Type A Behavior and Your Heart.* New York, NY: Fawcett, 1974.

Kerner, F. *Stress and Your Heart.* New York, NY: Hawthorne Books, 1961.

Kraus, H., and Raab, W. *Hypokinetic Disease.* Springfield, IL: Charles C Thomas, 1961.

McQuade, W., and Ailman, A. *Stress.* New York, NY: E. P. Dutton and Co., Inc., 1974.

Selye, H. *The Stress of Life.* New York, NY: McGraw-Hill, 1956.

Selye, H. *Stress Without Distress.* Philadelphia, PA: J. P. Lippincott, 1974.

Phase II

Bennett, A. *How to Live on 24 Hours a Day.* New York, NY: Corner Stone, 1962.

Drucker, P. *The Effective Executive.* New York, NY: Harper & Row, 1967.

Lakein, A. *How to Get Control of Your Time and Your Life.* New York, NY: Signet, 1973.

Mackenzie, R. A. *The Time Trap.* New York, NY: McGraw-Hill, 1972.

Webber, R. A. *Time and Management.* New York, NY: Van Nostrand, Rein-
hold, 1977.

Phase III
Benson, H. *The Relaxation Response.* New York, NY: William Morrow, 1976.
Dyer, W. *The Sky's the Limit.* New York, NY: Simon & Schuster, 1980.
Jacobson, E. *Progressive Relaxation.* Chicago, IL: The University of Chicago
Press, Midway Reprint, 1974.
Pelletier, K. *Mind as Healer, Mind as Slayer.* New York, NY: Dell, 1977.

Selected References for Three Phase Plan for Enjoying Fitness

Aerobic Fitness

Phase I
Allsen, P. E.; Harrison, J. M.; and Vance, B. *Fitness for Life.* Dubuque, IA:
William C. Brown Co., 1976.
Cooper, K. H. *The Aerobics Way.* New York, NY: M. Evans, 1977.
deVries, H. *Vigor Regained.* Englewood Cliffs, NJ: Prentice-Hall, 1974.
Kuntzleman, C. *The Exerciser's Handbook.* Spring Arbor, MI: Arbor Press,
1978.
Kuntzleman, C. *The Complete Book of Walking.* Skokie, IL: Publications
International (Consumer Guide), 1978.

Phase II
Fixx, J. *The Complete Book of Running.* New York, NY: Random House,
1977.
Glover, B., and Shepherd, J. *The Runner's Handbook.* New York, NY: The
Viking Press, 1977.
Kuntzleman, B. *The Complete Guide to Aerobic Dancing.* Skokie, IL: Publica-
tions International (Consumer Guide), 1980.
Ullyot, J. *Women's Running.* Mountain View, CA: World Publishers, 1976.

Phase III
Kostrubala, T. *The Joy of Running.* Philadelphia, PA: J. P. Lippincott, 1976.
Kuntzleman, C. *Rating the Exercises.* Skokie, IL: Publications International
(Consumer Guide), 1978.
Mitchell, C. *The Perfect Exercise.* New York, NY: Simon & Schuster, 1976.

Myers, C. R. *The Official YMCA Physical Fitness Handbook.* New York, NY: Popular Library, 1975.

Flexibility
Phase I
Uram, P. *The Complete Stretching Book.* Mountain View, CA: Anderson World, 1980.
Phase II
Anderson, B. *Stretching.* PO Box 2734, Fullerton, CA 92633.
Phase III
Devi, I. *Yoga for Americans.* New York, NY: New American Library, 1968.
Hittleman, R. *Introduction to Yoga.* New York, NY: Bantam Books, 1975.

Selected References for Three Phase Plan for Eating for Energy

Phase I
Berland, T. *Rating the Diets.* Skokie, IL: Publications International (Consumer Guide), 1978.
Deutsch, R. *Realities of Nutrition.* Palo Alto, CA: Bull Publishing, 1976.
Deutsch, R. *The Family Guide to Better Food and Better Health.* New York, NY: Bantam Books, 1979.
Food. A government publication that may be ordered from The Consumer Information Center, Dept. A., Pueblo, CO 81009.
Mayer, J. *A Diet for Living.* New York, NY: David H. McKay, 1975.
Pritikin, N. *The Pritikin Permanent Weight-Loss Manual.* New York, NY: Grosset & Dunlap, 1981.
Yudkin, J. *Sweet and Dangerous.* New York, NY: Bantam Books, 1973.
Phase II
American Heart Association Cookbook. New York, NY: Ballantine, 1977.
Connor, W. E.; Connor, S. L.; Fry, M. M.; and Warner, S. L. *The Alternative Diet Book.* Iowa City, IA: Department of Publications and Printing Service, The University of Iowa, 1976.
Keys, A., and Keys, M. *The Benevolent Bean.* New York, NY: Farrar, Straus, and Giroux, 1972.

Keys, A., and Keys, M. *How to Eat Well and Stay Well the Mediterranean Way*. New York, NY: Doubleday, 1975.

Lappe, F. M. *Diet for a Small Planet*. New York, NY: Ballantine, 1975.

Thomas, A. *The Vegetarian Epicure*. New York, NY: Vintage, 1972.

Phase III

Ewald, E. B. *Recipes for a Small Planet*. New York, NY: Ballantine, 1975.

Feingold, B. F. *Why Your Child Is Hyperactive*. New York, NY: Random House, 1975.

Jordan, J. *Wings of Life: Whole Vegetarian Cookery*. New York, NY: Crossing Press, 1976.

Lappe, F. M., and Ewald, E. B. *Great Meatless Meals*. New York, NY: Ballantine, 1974.

Schroeder, H. A. *The Trace Elements in Man*. Old Greenwich, CT: Devin-Adair Co., 1973.

Williams, R. *Nutrition against Disease*. New York, NY: Bantam Books, 1973.

Selected References for Three Phase Plan for Slimming

Phase I—Recommended Readings
Berland, T. *Rating the Diets*. Skokie, IL: Publications International, (Consumer Guide), 1978.

Kuntzleman, C. *The Activetics Alternative*. Spring Arbor, MI: Arbor Press, 1981.

Mayer, J. *Overweight: Cost, Causes and Control*. Englewood Cliffs, NJ: Prentice-Hall, 1968.

Phase II—Recommended Readings
Bailey, C. *Fit or Fat*. PO Box 23572, Pleasant Hill, CA 94523

Cooper, M. and Cooper, K. *Aerobics for Women*. New York, NY: M. Evans and Co., 1972.

Jordan, H., et al. *Eating is Okay!*. New York, NY: Rawson Associates Publishers, 1977.

Phase III—Recommended Readings
Beller, A. S. *Fat and Thin*. New York, NY: Farrar, Straus, and Giroux, 1977.

Konishi, F. *Exercise Equivalents of Foods*. Carbondale, IL: Southern Illinois University Press, 1973.

Selected References for Three Phase Plan for Relating to Others

Phase I
Augsburger, D. *Caring Enough to Confront*. Glendale, CA: Regal Books, 1976.
Fromm, E. *The Art of Loving*. New York, NY: Harper & Row, 1956.
Menninger, K. *The Vital Balance*. New York, NY: Viking Press, 1963.
Miller, W. R., and Muñoz, R. F. *How to Control Your Drinking*. Englewood Cliffs, NJ: Prentice-Hall, 1976.
Newman, M., and Berkowitz, B. *How to Be Your Own Best Friend*. New York, NY: Random House, 1971.
Newman, M., and Berkowitz, B. *How to Be Awake and Alive*. New York, NY: Random House, 1975.

Phase II
Calhoun, L. G. *Dealing with Crisis*. Englewood Cliffs, NJ: Prentice-Hall, 1976.
Caplan, F., ed. *The Parenting Advisor*. Garden City, NY: Anchor Press, 1978.
Dodson, F. *How to Parent*. Los Angeles, CA: Nash, 1970.
Ginott, H. *Between Parent and Child*. New York, NY: MacMillan 1965.
Gordon, T. *Parent Effectiveness Training*. New York, NY: Peter Wyden, 1970.
Hall, F. S., and Hall, D. T. *The Two Career Couple*. Reading, MA: Addison-Wesley, 1979.

Phase III
Akmakjian, H. *The Natural Way to Raise a Healthy Child*. New York, NY: Praeger, 1975.
Bach, G. R., and Deutsch, R. M. *Pairing*. New York, NY: Avon, 1975.
Howard, J. *Families*. New York, NY: Simon & Schuster, 1978.
Seidenberg, R. *Marriage between Equals*. Garden City, NY: Anchor Press, 1973.

Index